O. E. Akilov (Ed.)

Cutaneous Lymphomas: **Unusual Cases**　3

O. E. AKILOV (ED.)

Cutaneous Lymphomas
Unusual Cases 3

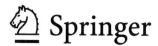

Editor
OLEG E. AKILOV
Cutaneous Lymphoma Program, Department of Dermatology
University of Pittsburgh
Pittsburgh, PA
USA

ISBN 978-3-030-59131-1   ISBN 978-3-030-59129-8   (eBook)
DOI 10.1007/978-3-030-59129-8

This Springer imprint is published by the registered company Springer Nature Switzerland AG
The registered company address is: Gewerbestrasse 11, 6330 Cham, Switzerland

Preface

Like the first two volumes, this book is a collection of cases with unusual clinical or pathological presentations of cutaneous lymphomas. Being rare in the practice of dermatologists and oncologists, cutaneous lymphomas are quite heterogeneous in their appearance and nature. For that reason, differential diagnostics is never straightforward. Particularly challenging is to establish the correct diagnosis in unusual cases, when something does not fit the classic pattern. The cases for this collection were carefully selected and provided by the experts in the field of cutaneous lymphomas from different countries. The concise format of cases along with short comments, outstanding clinical and histopathological illustrations, and carefully selected references was kept for consistency with the first two volumes.

Pittsburgh, PA, USA   OLEG E. AKILOV
July 2020

Contents

IV Extranodal NK/T-Cell Lymphoma

V γ/δ-Positive T-Cell Lymphomas

VI   CD8+ Cytotoxic Lymphoma and Mimickers

VII   Peripheral T-Cell Lymphoma with Secondary Skin Involvement

VIII   Posttransplant Lymphoproliferative Disorders

IX   Cutaneous B-Cell Lymphomas

X   Blastic Plasmacytoid Dendritic Cell Neoplasm

List of Authors

FARAH ABDULLA, MD
Beckman Research Institute, City of Hope
Cancer Center, Duarte, CA, USA
e-mail: fabdulla@coh.org

NIDHI AGGARWAL, MD
Department of Pathology, University of
Pittsburgh, Pittsburgh, PA, USA
e-mail: aggarwala@upmc.edu

OLEG E. AKILOV, MD, PhD
Cutaneous Lymphoma Program,
Department of Dermatology, University of
Pittsburgh, Pittsburgh, PA, USA
e-mail: akilovoe@upmc.edu

E. AKUFO-TETTEH, MD
Department of Dermatology, University
Hospital Birmingham, Birmingham, UK
e-mail: Emily.Akufo-Tetteh@uhb.nhs.uk

MARTINE BAGOT, MD, PhD
Department of Dermatology, APHP,
Saint-Louis Hospital, Université de Paris,
Paris, France
e-mail: martine.bagot@aphp.fr,
martine.bagot@gmail.com

MAXIME BATTISTELLA, MD, PhD
Department of Pathology, APHP,
Saint-Louis Hospital, Université de Paris,
Paris, France
e-mail: maxime.battistella@aphp.fr

IREN E. BELOUSOVA, MD, PhD
Department of Dermatology, Military
Medical Academy, Saint Petersburg, Russia
e-mail: irena.belousova@mail.ru

CLARA BERTUZZI, MD
Unit of Hematopathology, Department of
Experimental, Diagnostic and Specialty
Medicine, University of Bologna, Bologna,
Italy
e-mail: clarabertuzzi@gmail.com

AMINA BOUGRINE, MD
Department of Dermatology, Center for
Cutaneous Oncology, Brigham and
Women's Hospital, Dana-Farber Cancer
Institute, Harvard Medical School,
Boston, MA, USA
e-mail: amina.bougrine@gmail.com

PAULINE BRICE, MD
Department of Hematological Oncology,
APHP, Saint-Louis Hospital,
Paris, France
e-mail: pauline.brice@aphp.fr

MARIE-CHARLOTTE BRÜGGEN, MD, PhD
Department of Dermatology, University
Hospital Zurich, Zurich, Switzerland
e-mail: marie-charlotte.brueggen@usz.ch

A. N. BUI, BA
Harvard Medical School, Boston, MA,
USA
e-mail: Ai-Tram_Bui@hms.harvard.edu

SRIDHAR CHAGANTI, MD, PhD, MRCP,
FRCPATH Centre for Clinical
Hematology, University Hospital
Birmingham, NHS Foundation Trust,
Birmingham, UK
e-mail: Sridhar.Chaganti@uhb.nhs.uk

JISUN CHA, MD
Department of Dermatology and
Cutaneous Biology, Thomas Jefferson
University, Philadelphia, PA, USA
e-mail: Jisun.Cha@jefferson.edu

SONAL CHOUDHARY, MD
Department of Dermatology, University of
Pittsburgh, Pittsburgh, PA, USA
e-mail: choudharys@upmc.edu

MARY KAY COLLINS, MD
Department of Dermatology, University of
Pittsburgh, Pittsburgh, PA, USA
e-mail: collinsm3@upmc.edu

JADE CURY-MARTINS, MD, PhD
Department of Dermatology, University of
São Paulo, São Paulo, Brazil
e-mail: jadecury@yahoo.com.br

DAVID J. DICAUDO, MD
Department of Dermatology, Mayo Clinic,
Scottsdale, AZ, USA

FLORENTIA DIMITRIOU, MD
Department of Dermatology, University
Hospital Zurich, Zurich, Switzerland
e-mail: Florentia.Dimitriou@usz.ch

GOBOR DOBOS, MD, PhD
Department of Dermatology, APHP,
Saint-Louis Hospital, Université de Paris,
Paris, France
e-mail: gaborxdobos@gmail.com

M. DOERSCHNER
Department of Dermatology, University
Hospital Zurich, Zurich, Switzerland

VALERIA EVANGELISTA, MD
Unit of Dermatology, Department of
Experimental, Diagnostic and Specialty
Medicine, University of Bologna, Bologna,
Italy
e-mail: valeria.evangelista4@studio.unibo.it

TATYANA FELDMAN, MD
Lymphoma Division, John Theurer Cancer
Center, Hackensack University Medical
Center, Hackensack, NJ, USA
e-mail: tatyana.feldman@
hackensackmeridian.org

DAVID C. FISHER, MD
Dana-Farber/Brigham and Women's
Cancer Center, Harvard Medical School,
Boston, MA, USA
e-mail: david_c_fisher@dfci.harvard.edu

LARISA J. GESKIN, MD
Comprehensive Cutaneous Oncology
Center, Department of Dermatology,
Columbia University, Irving Medical
Center, New York, NY, USA
e-mail: ljg2145@cumc.columbia.edu

EMMANUELLA GUENOVA, MD,
PhD Department of Dermatology,
Lausanne University Hospital (CHUV),
University of Lausanne, Lausanne,
Switzerland
e-mail: emmanuella.guenova@unil.ch,
emmanuella.guenova@usz.ch

ALBA GUGLIELMO, MD
Dermatology Unit, Department of
Experimental, Diagnostic and Specialty
Medicine, University of Bologna, Bologna,
Italy
e-mail: albaguglielmo@gmail.com

CHRISTOPHER B. HERGOTT, MD,
PhD Department of Pathology, Brigham
and Women's Hospital, Boston, MA, USA
e-mail: chergott@partners.org

YE LIN HOCK, MD
Department of Histopathology, Walsall
Hospitals NHS Trust, Walsall, UK
e-mail: YeLin.Hock@uhb.nhs.uk

JONHAN HO, MD
Dermatopathology Unit, Department of
Dermatology, University of Pittsburgh,
Pittsburgh, PA, USA
e-mail: hoxxjx@UPMC.EDU

ARHTUR HUEN, MD, PhD
Department of Dermatology, University of
Pittsburgh, Pittsburgh, PA, USA
e-mail: huenac@upmc.edu

VICTORIA HUMPHREY, BS
University of Pittsburgh, School of
Medicine, Pittsburgh, PA, USA
e-mail: Humphrey.Victoria@medstudent.
pitt.edu

LINA HUSEINZAD, MD
Department of Dermatology, University of
Pittsburgh, Pittsburgh, PA, USA
e-mail: husienzadl@upmc.edu

JAROSLAW JEDRYCH, MD
Department of Dermatology, John Hopkins
University, Baltimore, MD, USA
e-mail: jjarosl2@jh.edu

VIKOTRYIA KAZLOUSKAYA, MD,
PhD Dermatopathology Unit, Department
of Dermatology, University of Pittsburgh,
Pittsburgh, PA, USA
e-mail: kazlouskayav@upmc.edu

WERNER KEMPF, MD
Department of Dermatology, University
Hospital Zürich, Kempf and Pfaltz
Histological Diagnostics, Zürich,
Switzerland
e-mail: werner.kempf@kempf-pfaltz.ch

Marios Koumourtzis, MD
2nd Department of Dermatology-
Venereology, ATTIKON University
Hospital, National and Kapodistrian
University of Athens Medical School,
Athens, Greece
e-mail: marioskoum@hotmail.com

Andrew A. Lane, MD, PhD
Department of Medical Oncology,
Dana-Farber Cancer Institute, Boston, MA,
USA
e-mail: andrew_lane@dfci.harvard.edu

Cecilia Larocca, MD
Department of Dermatology, Center for
Cutaneous Oncology, Brigham and
Women's Hospital, Dana-Farber Cancer
Institute, Harvard Medical School, Boston,
MA, USA
e-mail: CLAROCCA@BWH.HARVARD.
EDU

Nicole R. LeBoeuf, MD, MPH
Department of Dermatology, Brigham and
Women's Hospital, Center for Cutaneous
Oncology, Boston, MA, USA

Department of Dermatology, Dana-
Farber/Brigham and Women's Cancer
Center, Boston, MA, USA
E-MAIL: nleboeuf@bwh.harvard.edu

Jonathan J. Lee, MD
Department of Dermatology, Brigham
and Women's Hospital, Boston, MA,
USA
e-mail: Jonjlee1@gmail.com

Ivan V. Litvinov, MD, PhD, FRCPC
Division of Dermatology, McGill
University Health Centre, Montreal, QC,
Canada
e-mail: ivan.litvinov@mcgill.ca

Andrew Liu, BS
Department of Dermatology, University of
Pittsburgh, Pittsburgh, PA, USA
e-mail: liu.andrew@medstudent.pitt.edu

Xiao Xiao Li, MD
Department of Dermatology, University of
Pittsburgh, Pittsburgh, PA, USA
e-mail: lix20@upmc.edu

Cynthia Magro, MD
Department of Pathology, Weill Cornell
Medical Center, New York, NY, USA
e-mail: cym2003@med.cornell.edu

Helen Ma, MD
Department of Hematology & Oncology,
Columbia University Medical Center,
New York, NY, USA
e-mail: hm2715@cumc.columbia.edu

Aaron Mangold, MD
Department of Dermatology, Mayo Clinic,
Scottsdale, AZ, USA
e-mail: Mangold.Aaron@mayo.edu

Leonidas Marinos, MD
Hematopathology Department,
Evangelismos Hospital, National and
Kapodistrian University of Athens Medical
School, Athens, Greece
e-mail: lestrand@yahoo.gr

Xochiquetzal U. Martinez, MD
Division of Dermatology, Cutaneous
Lymphoma Program, City of Hope Cancer
Center, Beckman Research Institute,
Duarte, Duarte, CA, USA
e-mail: xomartinez@coh.org

Adelle de Masson, MD, PhD
Department of Dermatology, APHP,
Saint-Louis Hospital, Université de Paris,
Paris, France
e-mail: adele.demasson@aphp.fr

Martha Matsumoto, MD
Department of Dermatology, University of
Pittsburgh, Pittsburgh, PA, USA
e-mail: matsumotom@upmc.edu

Rutger C. Melchers, MD
Department of Dermatology, Leiden
University Medical Center, Leiden,
The Netherlands

David Michonneau, MD, PhD
Department of Hematological Oncology,
APHP, Saint-Louis Hospital, Paris, France
e-mail: david.michonneau@aphp.fr

Kevin Molloy, MD
Department of Dermatology, University
Hospital Birmingham, Birmingham, UK
e-mail: kevin.molloy1@nhs.net

Neda Nikbakht, MD, PhD
Department of Dermatology and
Cutaneous Biology, Thomas Jefferson
University, Philadelphia, PA, USA
e-mail: Neda.Nikbakht@jefferson.edu

MEGAN O'DONNELL, BS
Department of Dermatology and
Cutaneous Biology, Thomas Jefferson
University, Philadelphia, PA, USA
e-mail: Megan.O'Donnell@jefferson.edu

ROSANNE OTTEVANGER, MD
Department of Dermatology, Leiden
University Medical Center, Leiden,
The Netherlands

EVANGELIA PAPADAVID, MD, PhD
2nd Department of Dermatology-
Venereology, ATTIKON University
Hospital, National and Kapodistrian
University of Athens Medical School,
Athens, Greece
e-mail: papadavev@yahoo.gr

REGIS PEFFAULT DE LATOUR, MD, PhD
Department of Hematological Oncology,
APHP, Saint-Louis Hospital, Paris, France
e-mail: regis.peffaultdelatour@aphp.fr

ALESSANDRO PILERI, MD, PhD
Dermatology Unit, Department of
Experimental, Diagnostic and Specialty
Medicine, University of Bologna, Bologna,
Italy
e-mail: alessandropileri@hotmail.it

CHRISTIANE QUERFELD, MD, PhD
Division of Dermatology, Cutaneous
Lymphoma Program, Beckman Research
Institute, City of Hope Cancer Center,
Duarte, CA, USA
e-mail: cquerfeld@coh.org

KOEN D. QUINT, MD, PhD
Department of Dermatology, Leiden
University Medical Center, Leiden,
The Netherlands
e-mail: K.D.Quint@lumc.nl

CAROLINE RAM-WOLFF, MD
Department of Dermatology, APHP,
Saint-Louis Hospital, Paris, France
e-mail: caroline.ram-wolff@sls.aphp.fr

SREEJATA RAYCHAUDHURI, MD
Department of Internal Medicine,
University of Pittsburgh Medical Center,
McKeesport, PA, USA
e-mail: sreejata1@gmail.com

BETHANIE ROOKE, MD
Department of Dermatology, University
Hospital Birmingham, Birmingham, UK
e-mail: bethanie.rooke@nhs.net

ALLISON ROSENTHAL, DO
Division of Hematology/Oncology, Mayo
Clinic, Phoenix, AZ, USA
e-mail: srosen@coh.org

STEVE ROSEN
Beckman Research Institute, City of Hope
Cancer Center, Duarte, CA, USA

JOSE ANTONIO SANCHES, MD, PhD
Department of Dermatology, University of
São Paulo, São Paulo, Brazil
e-mail: jasanchesjr@gmail.com

AHMED SAWAS, MD
Department of Hematology & Oncology,
Columbia University Medical Center,
New York, NY, USA
e-mail: as4386@cumc.columbia.edu

JULIA SCARISBRICK, MBChB, MD
Department of Dermatology, University
Hospital Birmingham, Birmingham, UK
e-mail: Julia.Scariscbrick@uhb.nhs.uk

KEVIN J. SEVERSON, MD
Department of Dermatology, Mayo Clinic,
Scottsdale, AZ, USA
e-mail: Severson.Kevin@mayo.edu

SANMINDER SINGH, MD
Department of Dermatology, University of
Pittsburgh, Pittsburgh, PA, USA
e-mail: singhs8@upmc.edu

ANDREA M. STEVENS, MD
Department of Oncology, University
Hospital Birmingham, Birmingham, UK
e-mail: Andrea.Stevens@uhb.nhs.uk

STEVEN SWERDLOW, MD
Department of Pathology, University of
Pittsburgh, Pittsburgh, PA, USA
e-mail: swerdlowsh@upmc.edu

MEGAN H. TRAGER, BA
Department of Dermatology, Columbia
University Irving Medical Center,
New York, NY, USA
e-mail: mht2132@cumc.columbia.edu

CHARLES VAINDER, MD
Department of Dermatology, Cook County
Health, Chicago, IL, USA
e-mail: c.vainder@gmail.com

MARTEEN H. VERMEER, MD, PhD
Department of Dermatology, Leiden
University Medical Center, Leiden,
Netherlands
e-mail: m.h.vermeer@lumc.nl

BINDU VYDIANATH, MD
Department of Pathology, University
Hospital Birmingham, Birmingham, UK
e-mail: Bindu.Vydianath@uhb.nhs.uk

OLGA K. WEINBERG, MD
Department of Pathology, Boston
Children's Hospital, Boston, MA, USA
e-mail: Olga.Weinberg@
childrens.harvard.edu

REIN WILLEMZE, MD
Department of Dermatology, Leiden
University Medical Center, Leiden,
Netherlands
e-mail: rein.willemze@planet.nl

JINAH YOO, MD
Department of Dermatology, University
Hospital Birmingham, Birmingham, UK
e-mail: Jinah.Yoo@uhb.nhs.uk

JASMINE ZAIN, MD
Hematology and Hematopoietic Cell
Transplantation, T-Cell Lymphoma
Program, Beckman Research Institute, City
of Hope Cancer Center, Duarte, CA, USA
e-mail: jazain@coh.org

DAVIDE ZARDO, MD
Department of Pathology, University
Hospital Birmingham, Birmingham, UK
e-mail: Davide.Zardo@uhb.nhs.uk

Mycosis Fungoides

Mycosis fungoides, the most frequent cutaneous lymphoma, take many forms and can present with any primary morphological lesions. It has become a great masquerader in dermatology in the twenty-first century, taking syphilis in the nineteenth and twentieth centuries. Besides classic patches, plaques, and tumors, various atypical presentations are presented in the following cases. The epidermotropism with atypical lymphocytes at the dermo-epidermal junction is not limited to mycosis fungoides. Clinicopathological correlations should be helpful in those cases. Malignant lymphocytes possess skin-homing receptors that are getting lost in the advanced stage leading to the departure of cells into lymph nodes and blood. Loss of maturation markers such as CD5, CD7, and CD2 occur relatively early; when in later stages, de-differentiation is sometimes accompanied by the aberrant expression of unusual markers such as CD20, gamma delta, CD8 (double expression with CD4), and others. Metastatic spread to visceral organs remains to be extremely rare. For that reason, two cases of CNS involvement in two patients with tumors are of particular interest in this collection.

Case 1. Folliculotropic Mycosis Fungoides with Central Nervous System Involvement

F. Dimitriou, M. Doerschner, and E. Guenova

Age: 59   **Sex:** F

Clinical features: The patient presented with rapidly growing tumor on the right side of her chin and enlarged right submandibular lymph nodes without systemic symptoms. The skin biopsy showed folliculotropic atypical lymphocytes. Initially, a complete responds to LEBT, PUVA with IFN-α2a could be obsereved. Five months later, the patient presented with mild fatigue, personality changes, and difficulties of finding words. MRI showed brain metastasis of MF. The patient was treated with methotrexate and cytarabine, then thiotepa and carmustine followed by autologous HSCT.

Diagnosis: Folliculotropic mycosis fungoides, stage IIB (T3N1M0B0).

Follow-up: After complete response, the recurrence occurred 10 months after the autologous HSCT. Readministration of IFN-alfa-2a as maintenance treatment resulted in a durable complete remission.

Comment: The incidence of CNS involvement in MF is <1.3–1.6% in clinical studies and 10–15% in autopsy series. The risk of cerebral involvement is higher in cases with large-cell transformation, which was not detected in the present case. HSCT is a curative treatment option for advanced MF, with overall survival or relapse-free survival significantly longer in patients with allogeneic than with autologous SCT. Interestingly, in this case, readministration of IFN-alfa-2a as maintenance treatment after disease recurrence resulted in a durable complete remission.

References

Doerschner M, Pekar-Lukacs A, Messerli-Odermatt O, Dommann-Scherrer C, Rutti M, Muller AM, et al. Interferon alfa-2a maintenance after salvage autologous stem cell transplantation in atypical mycosis fungoides with central nervous system involvement. Br J Dermatol. 2019;181(6):1296–30.

Stein M, Farrar N, Jones GW, Wilson LD, Fox L, Wong RK, et al. Central neurologic involvement in mycosis fungoides: ten cases, actuarial risk assessment, and predictive factors. Cancer J. 2006;12(1):55–62.

Vu BA, Duvic M. Central nervous system involvement in patients with mycosis fungoides and cutaneous large-cell transformation. J Am Acad Dermatol. 2008;59(2 Suppl 1):S16–22.

Wu PA, Kim YH, Lavori PW, Hoppe RT, Stockerl-Goldstein KE. A meta-analysis of patients receiving allogeneic or autologous hematopoietic stem cell transplant in mycosis fungoides and Sezary syndrome. Biol Blood Marrow Transplant. 2009;15(8):982–90.

Fig. 1 Large tumor on the chin. Published with kind permission of The British Journal of Dermatology © Doerschner M et al 2019. All Rights Reserved

Fig. 2 Dense folliculotropic CD3+ CD4+ infiltrate of atypical cells. Published with kind permission of The British Journal of Dermatology © Doerschner M et al 2019. All Rights Reserved

Fig. 3 Magnetic resonance imaging (MRI) showing a CNS involvement with a T2 hyperintense lesion in the left frontal lobe before the autologous SCT, with complete response after autoSCT. Published with kind permission of The British Journal of Dermatology © Doerschner M et al 2019. All Rights Reserved

Fig. 4 Disease relapse after autoHSC

Fig. 5 Durable complete remission upon IFN-α-2a. Published with kind permission of The British Journal of Dermatology © Doerschner M et al 2019. All Rights Reserved

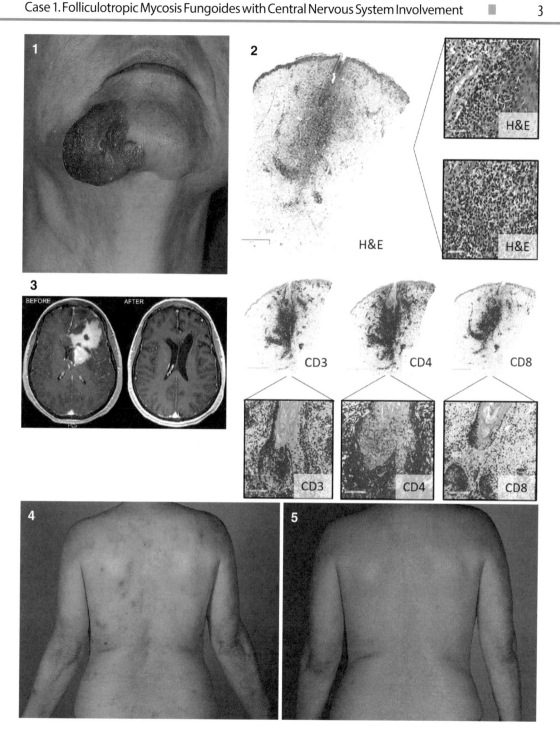

Case 2. Erythema Gyratum Repens-Like Mycosis Fungoides with Large Cell Transformation

A. Guglielmo, C. Bertuzzi, V. Evangelista, and A. Pileri

Age: 59   **Sex:**   F

Clinical features: A 3-year history of progressively growing annular to serpiginous erythematous patches and plaques on the trunk and limbs. The patient complained of itching, while her past medical history was unremarkable with no drug intake. Histology of a plaque showed an epidermotropic infiltrate consisting of atypical T-cells expressing CD3, CD4, CD45RO with CD7 loss. Fifteen to 20% of cells were large and expressed CD30+. No presence of fungi was detected.

Diagnosis: Erythema gyratum repens-like mycosis fungoides (EGR MF) with large cell transformation. Stage IB (T2bN0M0B0).

Follow-up: The patient has started the treatment with gemcitabine.

Comment: EGR MF is a rare variant of MF with only seven cases reported in the literature. Clinical presentation shows "wood-grained" serpiginous concentric erythematous lesions with fine scales at the top. In three cases, *T. rubrum* infection was observed and treatment with antifungals resolved the EGR-like features despite the persistence of MF patches and plaques. No fungal elements were found on biopsy in our patient. CD30+ large cell transformation in those cases is rare as indicated by a single report by Holcomb et al.

References

Cerri A, Vezzoli P, Serini SM, Crosti C, Berti E, Marzano AV. Mycosis fungoides mimicking erythema gyratum repens: an additional variant? Eur J Dermatol. 2010;20:540–1.

Holcomb M, Duvic M, Cutlan J. Erythema gyratum repens-like eruptions with large cell transformation in a patient with mycosis fungoides. Int J Dermatol. 2012;51:1231–3.

Jouary T, Lalanne N, Stanislas S, Vergier B, Delaunay M, Taïeb A. Erythema gyratum repens-like eruption in mycosis fungoides: is dermatophyte superinfection underdiagnosed in cutaneous T-cell lymphomas? J Eur Acad Dermatol Venereol. 2008;22:1276–8.

Moore E, McFarlane R, Olerud J. Concentric wood grain erythema on the trunk. Arch Dermatol. 2008;144:673–8.

Poonawalla T, Chen W, Duvic M. Mycosis fungoides with tinea pseudoimbricata owing totrichophyton rubrum infection. J Cutan Med Surg. 2006;10:52–6.

Fig. 1 Serpiginous erythematous patches and plaques on the limb

Fig. 2 Band-like infiltrate in the upper dermis

Fig. 3 Atypical lymphocytes in the upper dermis with admixture of the large cells

Fig. 4 Large cells are positive for CD30

Fig. 5 Atypical cells are positive for CD3

Fig. 6 Atypical cells are positive for CD4

Fig. 7 Loss of CD7 expression on atypical lymphocyte

Fig. 8 CD8 staining demonstrates the absence of CD8 expression on the atypical cells

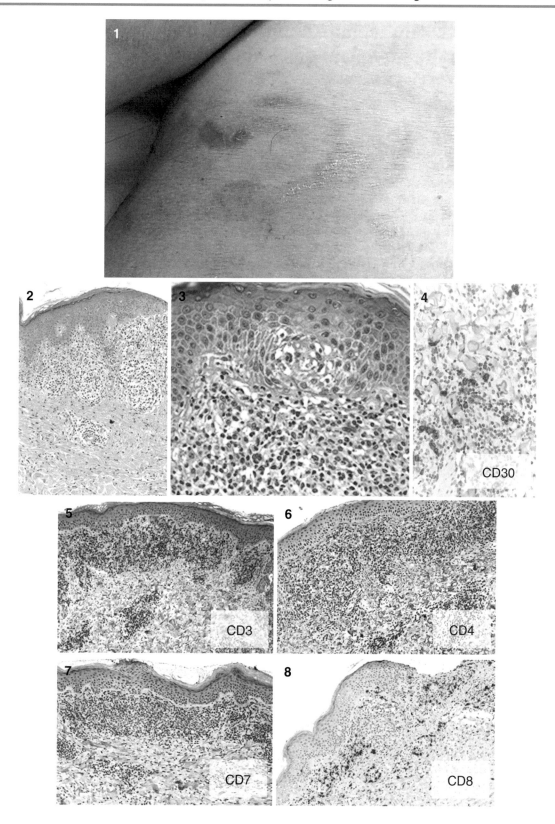

Case 3. Eczema Molluscatum in a Patient with Erythrodermic Mycosis Fungoides

L. Huseinzad, J. Ho, L. J. Geskin, and O. E. Akilov

Age: 41 **Sex:** F

Clinical features: The patient had a 14-year history of MF, stage IB (T2bN0M0B0) at the time of diagnosis. The patient previously failed topical steroids, nitrogen mustard, bexarotene, interferon-α, and ECP. Her MF slowly progressed until the patient became erythrodermic (stage IVA1, T4N1B1M0). The patient underwent four cycles of CHOP with total skin electron beam therapy. 1.5 months after numerous filiform papulopustules coalescing into sheets abruptly appeared on palms and soles and within weeks, diffusely covering the medial surfaces of both upper and lower extremities.

Diagnosis: Erythrodermic mycosis fungoides with secondary eczema molluscatum.

Follow-up: Oral bexarotene and weekly PEG-Interferon-α2a was initiated. The molluscum progressed despite 3 months of this treatment, and therapy was changed to romidepsin weekly infusions. No new papules of molluscum were noted at that time, but her MF continued to progress to extensive plaque and tumor involvement with recurrent infections. PET CT revealing worsening hilar lymphadenopathy and lung parenchymal involvement, for which pralatrexate was started. The patient continued to have recurring infections, worsening abdominal pain, and jaundice, with concern for lymphomatous involvement of the liver. She thereafter rapidly developed multifocal fungal pneumonia with refractory respiratory failure, hypotension, and altered mental status. She was eventually placed on comfort measures and passed away in the hospital, 20 months after the current presentation.

Comment: Molluscum contagiosum (MC) is a DNA poxvirus that causes classic umbilicated, pruritic skin lesions in children, sexually active adults, and immunosuppressed populations. MF patients have an increased risk of cutaneous infections by multiple mechanisms including extracutaneous lymphoma Additionally, patients with greater body surface area affected by MF and those with long-standing MF have a higher likelihood of infection.

Disseminated MC in patient with atopic dermatitis was previously attributed to the reduced Th1 activity with increased susceptibility to bacterial and viral infections, as evidenced by the frequent superimposed impetigo, eczema herpeticum, and eczema molluscatum. The similar mechanism can contribute to dissemination of MC in MF patients who have characteristic shift toward a Th2-cytokine profile with downregulation of the Th1 phenotype when MF progresses.

References

Le Treut C, Granel-Brocard F, Bursztejn A-C, Barbaud A, Plénat F, Schmutz J-L. Molluscum contagiosum surrounded by a white halo and Sezary syndrome. J Eur Acad Dermatol Venereol. 2015;29:1837–9.

Modschiedler K, Altenhoff J, Von Den Driesch P. Lymphoma molluscatum. Br J Dermatol. 2002;146:529–30.

Ohata C, Fukuda S, Hashikawa K, et al. Molluscum Contagiosum With CD30 + Cell Infiltration in a Patient With Mycosis Fungoides. Am J Dermatopathol. 2014;36:685–7.

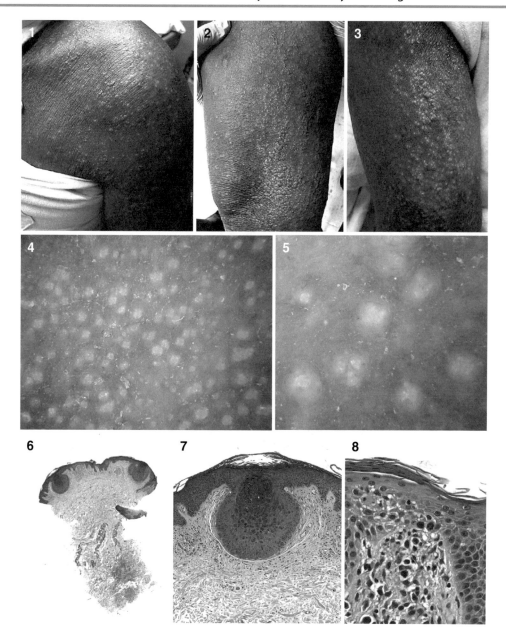

■ **Figs. 1–3** Filiform white papules of molluscum contagiosum (MC)

■ **Figs. 4–5** Dermatoscopic images of disseminated MC papules, ×2 (Fig. 4) and ×10 (Fig. 5)

■ **Fig. 6** Two MC papules. HE, ×2

■ **Fig. 7** Henderson-Patersen bodies, HE, ×10

■ **Fig. 8** Epidermotropic large atypical lymphocytes at dermo-epidermal junction. HE, ×10

Case 4. Parakeratosis Variegata-Like Poikilodermatous CD8+ Mycosis Fungoides

I. E. BELOUSOVA

Age: 54   **Sex:** F

Clinical features: The slow progression of hypo- and hyperpigmented patches and plaque gradually forming a network-like pattern since age of 25.

Diagnosis: Parakeratosis variegata-like poikilodermatous mycosis fungoides, stage IB (T2aN0M0B0).

Follow-up: Partial response to PUVA therapy. The patient lost to follow-up.

Comment: Poikilodermatous mycosis fungoides (PMF) is a variant of mycosis fungoides. Several similar conditions represent subvariants of PMF like poikiloderma vasculare atrophicans, parakeratosis (previosuly called "parapsoriasis") variegate (or "retiform parapsoriasis"), and mycosis fungoides-lichenoid type. Poikilodermic lesions characterized by alternating hypo- and hyperpigmentation, atrophy, and telangiectases. But not always all of those features present in the same patient. Sometimes lesions may become confluent to form bands and nets (reticular structures). The histopathology of the poikilodermatous mycosis fungoides is characterized by the presence of typical MF findings (e.g., the epidermotropism, atypia of lymphoid cells, loss of maturation markers), and may be accompanied by the interface, atrophy, and vascular changes. Seems like, the proportion of CD4+ and CD8+ cases are equal in PMF.

References

Dowling G, Freudenthal W. Dermatomyositis and poikiloderma atrophicans vascularis: a clinical and histological comparison. Br J Dermatol. 1938;50(10):519–39.

Kikuchi A, Naka W, Nishikawa T. Cutaneous T-cell lymphoma arising from parakeratosis variegata: long-term observation with monitoring of T-cell receptor gene rearrangements. Dermatology. 1995;190(2):124–7.

Samman PD. The natural history of parapsoriasis en plaques (chronic superficial dermatitis) and prereticulotic poikiloderma. Br J Dermatol. 1972;87(5):405–11.

Samman PD. Parkes Weber Lecture 1976. Mycosis fungoides and other cutaneous reticuloses. Clin Exp Dermatol. 1976;1(3):197–214.

Wätzig V, Roth H. [Parakeratosis variegata]. Dermatol Monatsschr. 1984;170(11):683–8.

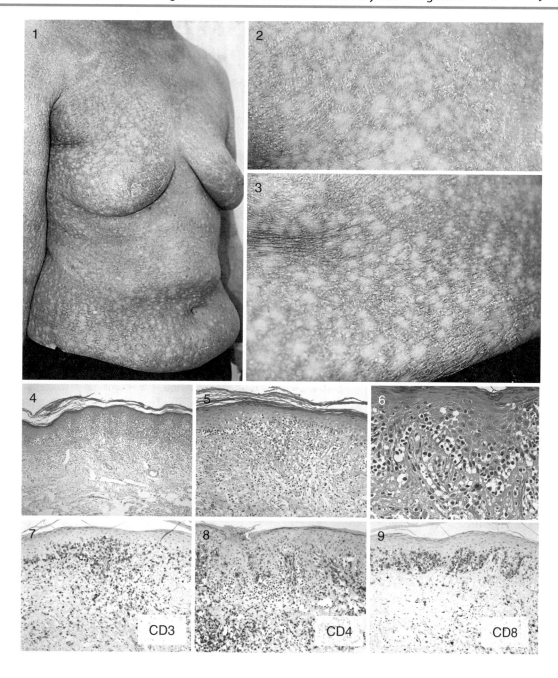

Fig. 1 Retiform confluent patches on the trunk

Figs. 2 and 3 Detailed network-like pattern of MF patches

Fig. 4 Band-like infiltrate of medium size atypical lymphocytes, HE

Fig. 5 Epidermostropism of atypical lymphocytes, HE

Fig. 6 Lymphocytes at the dermo-epidermal junction, HE

Fig. 7 Atypical cells are positive for CD3

Fig. 8 Admixture of reactive CD4 cells

Fig. 9 Positive CD8 staining of the epidermotropic lymphocytes

Case 5. Parakeratosis variegata in a patient with CD8+ mycosis fungoides with post-inflammatory hypopigmentation

L. Huseinzad, J. Ho, and O. E. Akilov

Age: 34   **Sex:** M

Clinical features: The patient with 8 year of history of itchy, scaly, hyperpigmented patches initially on the neck. Within a year, these patches generalized to involve the chest, back, abdomen, arms, and legs. No accompanying systemic symptoms. The current clinical exam with hyperpigmented papules coalescing into a net-like structure on the lower extremities bilaterally and hypopigmented and hyperpigmented scaly patches and plaques covering all. Laboratory and radiologic investigation were unrevealing. Histologic evaluation revealed extensive lymphocytic vacuolar interface and CD2+, CD3+, CD8+ lymphocyte exocytosis with diminished CD5 and CD7 staining as well as numerous dermal melanophages. Notably, after the resolution, the patches and plaque left hypopigmentation.

Diagnosis: Parakeratosis variegata in a patient with CD8+ mycosis fungoides, stage IB (T2bN0M0B0).

Follow-up: On methotrexate 20 mg orally weekly and topical steroids. Previously had failed PUVA and topical steroids in 2009, then had been off any treatment for 6 years during his incarceration, until re-establishing care in 2015. At that time, he improved with NB-UVB and bexarotene, but could not keep up with NB-UVB appointments and had to discontinue bexarotene due to severe muscle weakness.

Comment: Parakeratosis variegate (PV) was first described by Unna in 1890 as hyperpigmented lichenoid papules in a retiform array along with epidermal atrophy and telangiectasias PV can be seen in genodermatoses, connective tissue diseases, and in association with MF. The relationship of PV to MF remains controversial. PV has been reported to evolve from parapsoriasis and pityriasis lichenoides chronica, but even with pronounced epidermotropism and extensive cutaneous involvement may be reversible.

Our patient had PV secondary to long-standing CD8+ MF. Thus, we hypothesize that PV could be also a reaction pattern in predisposed individuals.

References

Choi MS, Lee JB, Kim SJ, Lee SC, Won YH, Yun SJ. A case of poikiloderma vasculare atrophicans. Ann Dermatol. 2011;23(Suppl 1):S48–52.

Mahajan VK, Chauhan PS, Mehta KS, Sharma AL. Poikiloderma vasculare atrophicans: a distinct clinical entity? Indian J Dermatol. 2015;60:216.

Rogoziński T, Zekanowski C, Kaldan L, Blaszczyk M, Majewski S, Jabłońska S. Parakeratosis variegata: a possible role of environmental hazards? Dermatology. 2000;201:54–7.

- **Fig. 1** Retiform coalescent papules on the posterior foreleg
- **Fig. 2** Ashy, hyperpigmented patches and plaque with postinflammatory hypopigmentation
- **Fig. 3** Sparse lymphocytic infiltrate. HE, ×10
- **Fig. 4** Highly atypical epidermotropic lymphocyte. HE. ×40
- **Fig. 5** CD3+ atypical lymphocytes
- **Fig. 6** Negative CD4 stain
- **Fig. 7** CD8+ atypical lymphocytes
- **Fig. 8** Diminished CD5 expression
- **Fig. 9** Diminished CD7 expression
- **Fig. 10** Ki-67 is not increased and positively stains 10–15% of CD3+ atypical lymphocytes

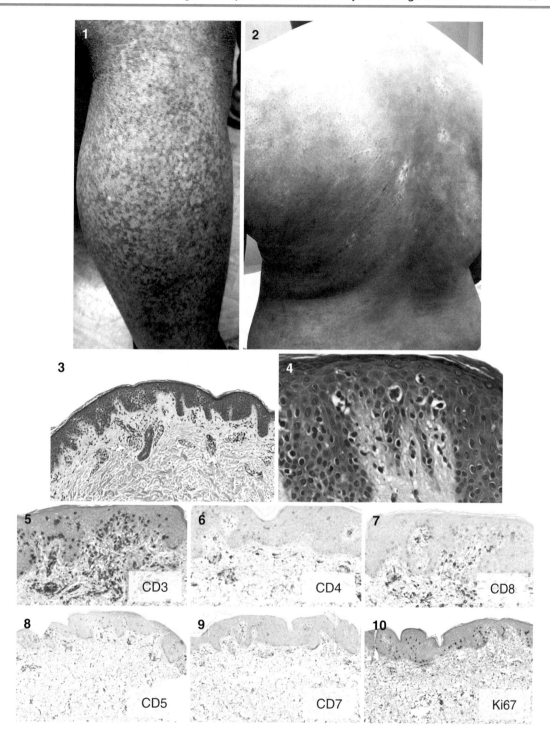

Case 6. Poikilodermatous Mycosis Fungoides

K. Molloy, B. Vydianath, D. Zardo, and J. Scarisbrick

Age: 59   **Sex:** F

Clinical features: An 18-month history of an intensely pruritic and painful burning rash which began on the chest. This slowly spread to cover most of her trunk, limbs, and scalp with associated alopecia. Physical examination showed widespread poikilodermatous reticulated erythematous patches affecting 60–70% body surface area becoming confluent on both lower limbs. This was accompanied by thickened fissured skin on the hands and generalized hair loss on the scalp with marked perifollicular scaling. The patient had received multiple treatments for a presumed diagnosis of a benign lichenoid dermatoses which included clobetasol propionate 0.05% ointment, oral prednisolone (30 mg daily), and subcutaneous methotrexate (15–20 mg weekly) with minimal response. No peripheral blood involvement was demonstrated by flow cytometry (CD4+ CD7−: 65.55 cells/mm^3 and CD4+ CD26−: 96.6 cell/mm^3) and serum lactate dehydrogenase level was elevated (265 U/L, normal 135–214 U/L). CT thorax, abdomen, and pelvis showed no evidence of lymphadenopathy. Skin histology showed lichenoid interface inflammation with epidermal atrophy, no loss of T-cell markers (CD3, CD2, CD5 and CD7), and a CD4:CD8 ratio of 3:1. The same T-cell clonal rearrangement was demonstrated in five separate skin biopsies.

Diagnosis: Poikilodermatous MF, stage IB (T2aN0M0B0).

Follow-up: The patient did not respond to NB UVB. Given a partial response to localized radiotherapy (8 Gy, 2 fractions) to the back of her hands, she was treated with total skin electron beam therapy (TSEBT). TSEBT (12 Gy in 8 fractions) was discontinued prematurely due to blistering eruption on both lower limbs but overall resulted in a partial response. The patient is now on cobomarsen (MRG-106, miR-155 inhibitor) with improved symptoms and without any adverse effects.

Comment: Poikilodermatous MF, also termed as poikiloderma vasculare atrophicans is a rare distinct clinicopathological variant of MF that more commonly presents in females and at a younger age. Histology may be inconclusive and in these cases the detection of the same T-cell clone in multiple biopsies confirmed the diagnosis. It is more frequently associated with lymphomatoid papulosis and in a greater proportion of cases CD8+ CD4− atypical lymphocytes appear to predominate. The overall prognosis appears to be favorable and there is a good response to phototherapy (Abbott et al. 2011). Interestingly, our patient had CD4+ phenotype and had no response to phototherapy. TSEBT appears to be a good therapeutic option for those patients with large body surface involvement who are refractory to phototherapy. The TSEBT protocol may need to be attenuated in these patients due to profound changes in their skin.

References

Abbott RA, Sahni D, Robson A, et al. Poikilodermatous mycosis fungoides: a study of its clinicopathological, immunophenotypic, and prognostic features. J Am Acad Dermatol. 2011;65:313–9.

Vasconcelos Berg R, Valente NYS, Fanelli C, et al. Poikilodermatous mycosis fungoides: comparative study of clinical, histopathological and immunohistochemical features. Dermatology. 2019:1–6.

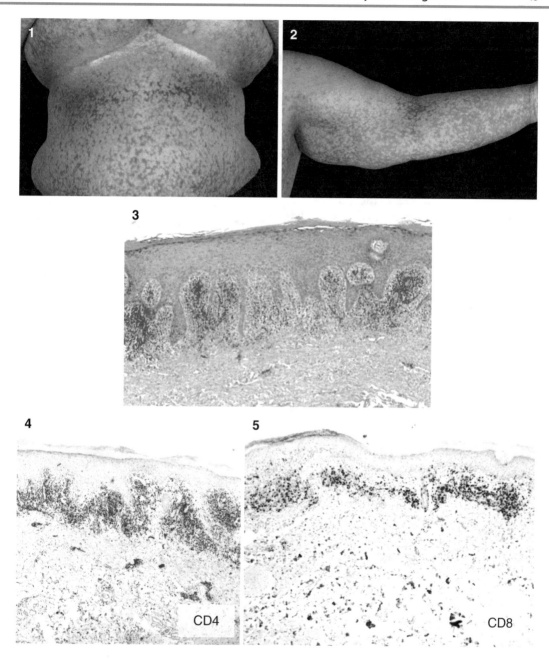

Fig. 1 Mottled hypo- and hyperpigmentary patches on anterior trunk

Fig. 2 Poikilodermatous reticulated erythematous patches on the upper limb

Fig. 3 Superficial dermal lichenoid lymphocytic infiltrate with interface inflammation with scattered apoptotic keratinocytes. HE, 10×

Fig. 4 CD4 expression of the infiltrating cells. 10×

Fig. 5 CD8 expression of the infiltrating cells. 10×

Case 7. Tumor Mycosis Fungoides with Xanthomatized Atypical Lymphocytes

V. Kazlouskaya, J. Ho, and O. E. Akilov

Age: 82   **Sex:** M

Clinical features: The patient with 4-year history of patches and plaque of MF covering 50–60% of body surface area, stage IB (T2bN0M0B0) at diagnosis. For 2 years, the patient was treated with topical steroid and oral methotrexate 25 mg PO weekly until he had started developing tumors. At the current presentation, there are large tumors with an eroded surface. The flow cytometry on the peripheral blood and bone marrow biopsy did not show the involvement by lymphoma. PET/CT scan demonstrated skin thickening in the abdominal wall as well as metabolic, not hypermetabolic axillary lymph node and mildly hypermetabolic left inguinal lymph node that has been resolved on the follow-up scan. Repeated biopsy from the tumor on the left lower back demonstrated mild acanthosis with epidermotropism and Pautrier microabscesses, as well as deep and diffuse dermal infiltrate with atypical lymphocytes without signs of large cell transformation and foamy cells with large amount of cytoplasm. Atypical cells expressed CD3, CD4, and CD5 with diminished expression of CD7. Few scattered cells expressed CD30 and CD20. Electron microscopy of the infiltrate demonstrated lipid inclusions in histiocytes. Adipophilin immunostain confirmed the presence of numerous lipid particles in the infiltrate.

Diagnosis: Mycosis fungoides, stage IIB (T3N1 M0B0) with xanthoma-like changes in the atypical cells.

Follow-up: Methotrexate was discontinued and the patient was started on pralatrexate. 14 months after biweekly doses and LEBT on tumors, the patient's MF was under control.

Comment: Presence of xanthomatous lipidized cells in the infiltrate of mycosis fungoides was previously described and may be clinically associated with co-existing hyperlipidemia. The pathogenesis of this phenomenon is not completely understood. It may present a degenerative process in old atypical lymphocytes in persistent plaques and tumors. The alternative explanation is that this is a result of histiocytic phagocytosis of lipid particles released by dying cells or transferred from highly lipidized blood in patients with hyperlipidemia. Lipid inclusions were documented in both histiocytes and atypical lymphocytes using electron microscopy. It is unclear if they have been diffused to a lymphocyte or have been synthesized. T cells have low density lipoprotein receptors and may participate in abnormal lipid accumulation similarly as it happens in atherosclerosis. Histopathology of such infiltrates may mimic xanthomatous or infection conditions, and caution in interpretation is needed.

Interestingly, our patient did not have hyperlipidemia. Unusually, his tumor with xanthomatized lymphocytes were limited to the one part of the body (left lower flank), did not spread, and were very resistant to therapy, persisting at one location for more than 2 years.

References

Ross EV, Roman I, Rushin JM, Cobb MW, Friedman KJ. Xanthomatized atypical T cells in a patient with mycosis fungoides and hyperlipidemia. Arch Dermatol. 1992;128:1499–502.

Tse K, Tse H, Siidney J, Sette A, Ley K. T cells in atherosclerosis. Int Immunol. 2003;25:615–22.

Winkler JK, Hoffmann J, Enk A, Toberer F. Diffuse plane xanthomas associated with mycosis fungoides. Hautarzt. 2009;70:438–42.

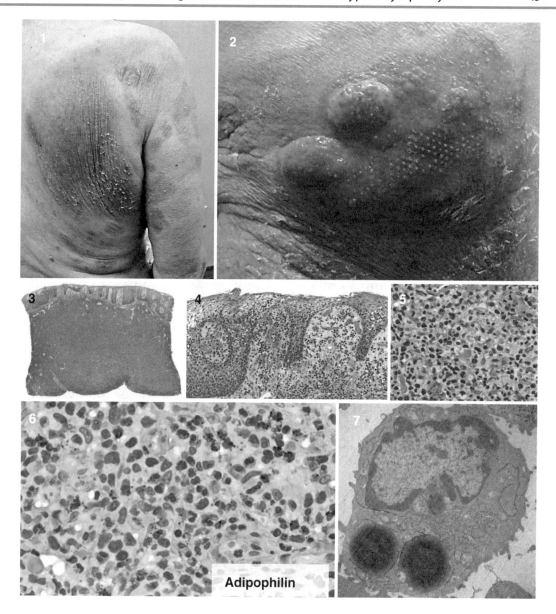

■ Fig. 1 Erythematous scaly patches and plaques on the trunk and upper extremities

■ Fig. 2 Close-up image of coalescing tumors on the left flank with yellowish hue

■ Fig. 3 Biopsy of the tumor mass demonstrating deep and diffuse infiltrate. HE, ×2. Published with kind permission of © Viktoryia Kazlouskaya 2019. All Rights Reserved

■ Fig. 4 Central ulceration of the top of the ulcer. HE, ×10. Published with kind permission of © Viktoryia Kazlouskaya 2019. All Rights Reserved

■ Fig. 5 Higher magnification showed the mixed infiltrate composed of foamy histiocytes, atypical lymphocytes, and eosinophils. Published with kind permission of © Viktoryia Kazlouskaya 2019. All Rights Reserved

■ Fig. 6 Adipophilin stain highlighting numerous fat granules in the atypical lymphocytes and histiocytes. Published with kind permission of © Viktoryia Kazlouskaya 2019. All Rights Reserved

■ Fig. 7 Electron microscopy of an atypical lymphocyte with convoluted nucleus with lipid granules

Case 8. CD20+ Mycosis Fungoides Partially Responsive to Rituximab

C. Vainder, J. Jedrych, J. Ho, and O. E. Akilov

Age: 72   **Sex:** M

Clinical features: The patient with a 21-year history of patches and plaque of MF, stage IB (T2bN0M0B0) at diagnosis. All that time, he was using only topical steroids and was overall satisfied with his disease control. At the current presentation, 50% of body surface area was occupied by erythematous plaques on the lower portion of trunk and upper thighs. Some plaques were covered with yellowish crusts. Systemic workup did not show any lymphoma involvement beyond the skin. Biopsy was performed and demonstrated mild hyperparakeratosis overlying a dense superficial band like, perivascular and interstitial infiltrate composed of lymphocytes with mildly enlarged hyperchromatic nuclei and irregular nuclear contour. The lymphoid infiltrate is predominately composed of CD3+ T cells without significant loss of CD2 but with diminished expression of CD5 and CD7. Those cells had aberrant CD20 expression, while the expression of other B cell markers such as CD79a, Pax-5, and Bcl-6 was negative.

Diagnosis: Mycosis fungoides, stage IB (T2bN0 M0B0) with aberrant CD20 expression.

Follow-up: The patient was started on rituximab and notice an improvement after 3 doses. However, no improvement was observed with the continuation of rituximab, and after fourth infusion, the medication was discontinued. The repeated biopsy did not show the aberrant expression of CD20+ on atypical T cells. The patient started romidepsin, achieved PR after 3 cycles, had less than 5% of body surface area occupied by patches and discontinued the treatment on his own. The patient lost follow-up for 2 years. During this time, he did not use any treatment. When he came back, he had 12% of body surface area occupied by patches, which he preferred to treat with NB UVB.

Comment: The aberrant expression of CD20 on T cells in mycosis fungoides has been reported previously. The most common hypotheses explaining this phenomenon are (1) the raise of malignant T cells from a CD20+ progenitor; (2) the acquisition of CD20 during the lymphoma progression and de-differentiation. We support the last one. The original diagnostic biopsy did not show CD20 positivity. Our patient had non-treated slowly progressing MF for 20 years. Most likely, that was the reason for the acquired CD20 expression. Another important observation is the inefficacy of rituximab for those patients. Despite some improvement initially, the response to rituximab in our patient was shortlived. The repeated biopsy did not show CD20 expression anymore, which also is in concordance with previous observations. According to the literature, CD20 expression on T cells indicates the worse prognosis. Several patients who had CD20+ MF died soon after diagnosis. Our patient is still alive, 2 years after, on skin-directed therapies only, which may be an exception rather than a rule in those cases.

Reference

Tschetter AJ, Zafar F, Moye MS, et al. CD20+ cutaneous T-cell lymphoma with phenotypic shift after treatment with rituximab: case report and review of the literature. JAAD Case Rep. 2020;6(4):308–10.

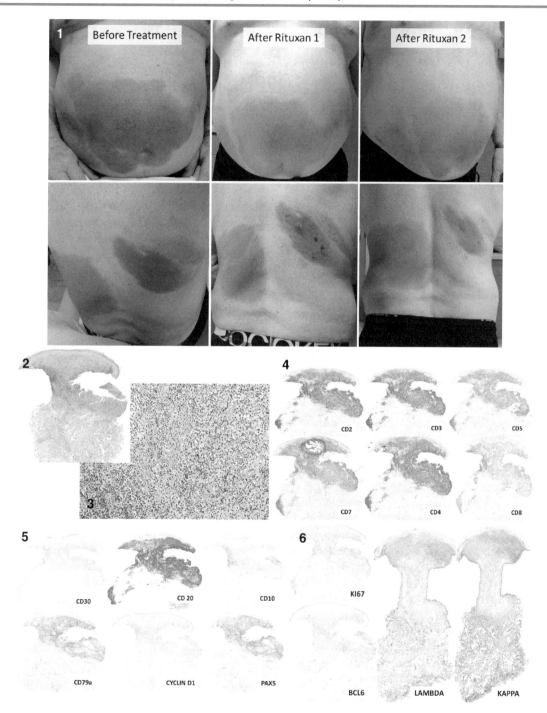

■ Fig. 1 Clinical pictures showing improvement of cutaneous plaques after rituximab

■ Fig. 2 Deep and dense lymphocytic infiltrate occupying all dermis. HE, ×2

■ Fig. 3 Small and medium sized lymphocytes predominate in the infiltrate. HE, ×10

■ Fig. 4 The majority of lymphocytes are CD2+ CD3+ CD4+ with diminished expression of CD5 and CD7

■ Fig. 5 Strong CD20 expression on CD3+ lymphocytes with negative CD79a and Pax-5

■ Fig. 6 Ki-67 is not increased. No κ or λ restriction

Case 9. Chronic Lymphocytic Inflammation with Pontine Perivascular Enhancement Responsive to Steroids (CLIPPERS) in a Patient with Granulomatous Mycosis Fungoides and Multiple Tumors

J. Lee, J. Jedrych, J. Ho, and O. E. Akilov

Age: 60 **Sex:** M

Clinical features: The patient presented with a 6-month history of patches, plaques, and tumors on his buttocks, back, and extremities associated with fatigue but no weight loss or night sweats. Based on the clinical, pathologic, and radiographic findings, a diagnosis of MF, stage IIB (T3N1M0B0) was made. The patient was started on pralatrexate 15 mg/m^2. After completion of 2 cycles, significant clinical improvement was noted, and the patient was transitioned to oral bexarotene. However, the patient's MF progressed within a month, and pralatrexate was re-started. Two weeks after, the patient presented to the Emergency Department with new-onset dysarthria. MRI of the brain revealed a 1.4 cm curvilinear, punctate, enhancing lesion on the right ventral-most aspect of the pons with surrounding vasogenic edema. Analysis of cerebrospinal fluid revealed a heterogeneous T-cell predominant lymphoplasmacytic population with atypical lymphocytosis. Chest, abdomen, and pelvis CT revealed no evidence of lymphadenopathy or any involvement of internal viscera. The patient was started on intravenous dexamethasone, with complete resolution of his neurologic symptoms and neuro-radiologic findings. The patient has been maintained on low dose prednisone without recurrence of his neurologic symptoms.

Diagnosis: Mycosis fungoides, stage IIB (T3N0 M0B0) with CLIPPERS.

Follow-up: The disease has rapidly progressed and patient developed tumors all over his body.

Nivolumab as well as 3 cycles of R-CHOP chemotherapy and palliative bendamustine were not effective. The patient received total body skin electron therapy, achieved CR and continues being in CR for the last 24 months.

Comment: CLIPPERS is an emerging, recently described lymphocytic inflammatory syndrome involving the brainstem. First described in 2010, CLIPPERS is typified clinically by acute to subacute neurologic symptoms referable to focal cerebral dysfunction (gait ataxia and diplopia as well as dysarthria, altered sensation and paresthesias of the face, dizziness, nystagmus, spastic paraparesis, sensory loss and pseudobulbar affect). Middle-aged adults are most commonly affected, and based on available reports there appears to be a slight male predominance. Isolated reports of CLIPPERS in association with other conditions have been reported: peripheral T-cell lymphoma, chronic hepatitis B infection, herpes zoster, B-cell lymphoma, and multiple sclerosis. To the best of the authors' knowledge, this is the first reported case of CLIPPERS syndrome occurring in association with MF.

References

Pittock SJ, et al. Chronic lymphocytic inflammation with pontine perivascular enhancement responsive to steroids (CLIPPERS). Brain. 2010;133(9):2626–34.

Taieb G, et al. Long-term outcomes of CLIPPERS (chronic lymphocytic inflammation with pontine perivascular enhancement responsive to steroids) in a consecutive series of 12 patients. Arch Neurol. 2012;69(7):847–55.

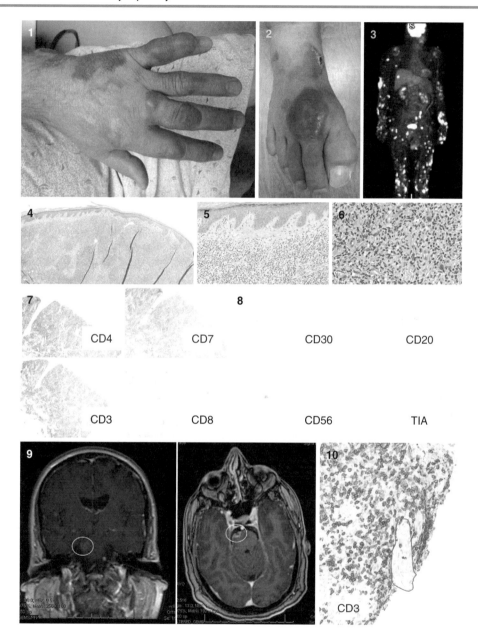

Fig. 1 Tumors on the left hand

Fig. 2 Tumors on the right foot

Fig. 3 PET scan showed multiple skin tumors but no visceral involvement

Fig. 4 Dense lymphocytic infiltrate, HE, ×2

Fig. 5 The Grenz zone and the absence of the epidermotropism. HE, ×20

Fig. 6 Mixed lympho-histiocytic infiltrate, HE, ×20

Fig. 7 The lymphocytes are positive for CD3, CD4, and CD7

Fig. 8 Negative stains for CD30, CD20, CD56, and TIA

Fig. 9 MRI brain showed 10.2 × 0.8 × 1.4 cm ring enhancing lesion in the right side of pons with vasogenic edema

Fig. 10 Neurotropism of CD3+ lymphocytes

Case 10. Folliculotropic Mycosis Fungoides with Exuberant Neutrophil-Rich Scale and Follicular Plugging Mimicking Hypertrophic Actinic Keratosis

V. Kazlouskaya, J. Ho, and O. E. Akilov

Age: 54   **Sex:** M

Clinical features: The patient presented with a 3-year history of a folliculotropic mycosis fungoides stage IB (T2bN0M0B0). The patient was initially well controlled on bexarotene but had to discontinue it due to chronic non-controllable hypercholesterolemia. After discontinuation of bexarotene, his MF progressed. Moreover, the patient developed new patches around his eyes with a thick hyperkeratotic adherent scale clinically similar to hypertrophic actinic keratosis (AK) or squamous cell carcinoma. Shave biopsy was performed and demonstrated significant hyperkeratosis with neutrophilic scale crust accompanied by follicular plugging. Follicular mucin depositions were absent. There was a band-like infiltrate composed of mildly atypical lymphocytes with significant epidermotropism and folliculotropism. T-cell receptor gene rearrangement showed a monoclonal pattern identical to one discovered initially.

Diagnosis: Folliculotropic mycosis fungoides with exuberant neutrophil-rich scale and follicular plugging mimicking hypertrophic AK.

Follow-up: Due to his MF progression, that patient has started biweekly pralatrexate infusions. His hyperkeratotic patches completely resolved after a single infusion of pralatrexate. Currently, after 10 cycles, the patient near 90% clear and remains to have a stable patch disease.

Comment: Histopathology of folliculotropic MF is often characterized by perifollicular infiltrates and mucinous degeneration of the follicle. Keratin plugging of the hair follicle without significant mucin deposits is seen in rare case. Occasionally, the epidermal changes may include follicular cystic changes, hyperplasia of the follicular epithelium, granulomatous inflammatory reaction secondary to ruptured hair follicles. Basaloid follicular lymphoid hyperplasia of the follicle with proliferations of epithelial cells extending from intact hair follicles was described previously. In our patient, follicular plugging was accompanied by thick hypertrophic scale clinically mimicking the hypertrophic AK. Since those hyperkeratotic patches completely responded to lymphoma-specific medication, we believe that hyperkeratosis was lymphocyte-driven. While the presence of AK is common in elderly and may co-exist in patients with MF, this unusual presentation may indicate the necessity of a biopsy to establish the diagnosis properly and to avoid incorrect treatment.

References

Bakar O, Seçkin D, Demirkesen C, Baykal C, Büyükbabani N. Two clinically unusual cases of folliculotropic mycosis fungoides: one with and the other without syringotropism. Ann Dermatol. 2004;26:385–91.

Gerami P, Guitart J. The spectrum of histopathologic and immunohistochemical findings in folliculotropic mycosis fungoides. Am J Surg Pathol. 2007;31:1430–8.

Marschalkó M, Erős N, Kontár O, Hidvégi B, Telek J, Hársing J, Jókai H, Bottlik G, Rajnai H, Szepesi Á, Matolcsy A, Kárpáti S, Csomor J. Folliculotropic mycosis fungoides: clinicopathological analysis of 17 patients. J Eur Acad Dermatol Venereol. 2015;29:964–72.

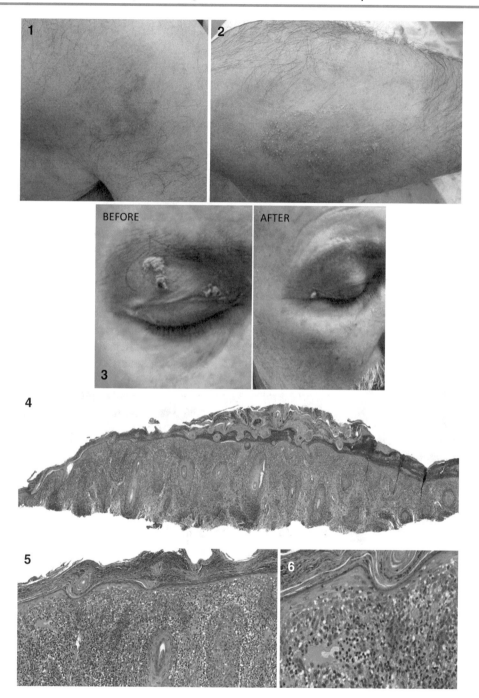

Fig. 1 Prominent follicular accentuation in the patch on the left chest at diagnosis

Fig. 2 A patch with pronounced follicular hyperkeratotic papules on the right elbow during the initial presentation

Fig. 3 Hyperkeratotic patches on the right upper eyelid and the right eyebrows mimicking hypertrophic AK before and after treatment with pralatrexate

Fig. 4 The unusual epidermal hyperplasia with prominent hyperkeratosis and follicular plugging and collections of neutrophils. HE, 2×

Fig. 5 Lichenoid epidermotropic and folliculotropic infiltrates under the area of hyperkeratosis

Fig. 6 The high magnification showing prominent epidermotropism

Case 11. Small plaque parapsoriasis-like mycosis fungoides

X. Li, V. Humphrey, J. Ho, and O. E. Akilov

Age: 67   Sex: M

Clinical features: The patient presented with a 1-year history of erythematous non-pruritic digitate well-defined coin-shaped patches on the flank only. The biopsy showed compact orthokeratosis and, in some areas, marked parakeratosis with serum deposition on the stratum corneum. The epidermis showed marked lymphocytic epidermotropism, spongiosis, and focal intraepithelial lymphocytes, together with vacuolar degeneration of the basal layer. The intraepithelial lymphocytes are hyperchromatic and have crenulated nuclear borders. Occasional dyskeratotic keratinocytes are identified, and there is dermal melanin deposition. The infiltrate is composed almost entirely of CD3-positive T cells. The T cells exhibit preserved staining for CD2 and CD5, while CD7 staining is slightly diminished. CD4:CD8 ratio is increased (~6:1). Ki-67 stain reveals a slightly increased proliferative index in the epidermotropic lymphoid infiltrate. Due to negative TCR gene rearrangement studies, the patient was diagnosed with small plaque parapsoriasis and treated with topical steroids as needed.

Six years later, the patient presented with classic patches on buttocks, while digitate patches on the flank disappear entirely. Thus, the diagnosis of the patch stage of MF was rendered based on typical clinical presentation and suggestive histology.

Diagnosis: Mycosis fungoides stage IA (T1aN0M0B0).

Follow-up: A staging workup was performed, showing no evidence of extracutaneous disease. The patient was not interested in any treatment options and lost follow-up.

Comment: This case illustrates that the early patch MF can be mistaken for a small plaque parapsoriasis. While classically, patch MF presents in a bathing-trunk distribution, the unusual presentation of patches on the flanks can create some confusion.

A biopsy is essential to differentiate between those two diseases. While small plaque parapsoriasis is a spongiotic process with parakeratosis, MF is characterized by the epidermal collections of neoplastic lymphocytes of atypical morphology.

Our patient initially exhibited clinical and morphological features of both diseases. The absence of a distinct TCR clone was supportive of small plaque parapsoriasis. However, several years later, the patient presented with classic patch MF presentation indication that long-term follow-up of these patients is necessary for proper care.

References

Baderca F, Chiticariu E, Baudis M, Solovan C. Biopsying parapsoriasis: quo vadis? Are morphological stains enough or are ancillary tests needed? Romanian J Morphol Embryol. 2014;55(3 Suppl):1085–92.

Haeffner AC, Smoller BR, Zepter K, Wood GS. Differentiation and clonality of lesional lymphocytes in small plaque parapsoriasis. Arch Dermatol. 1995;131(3):321–4.

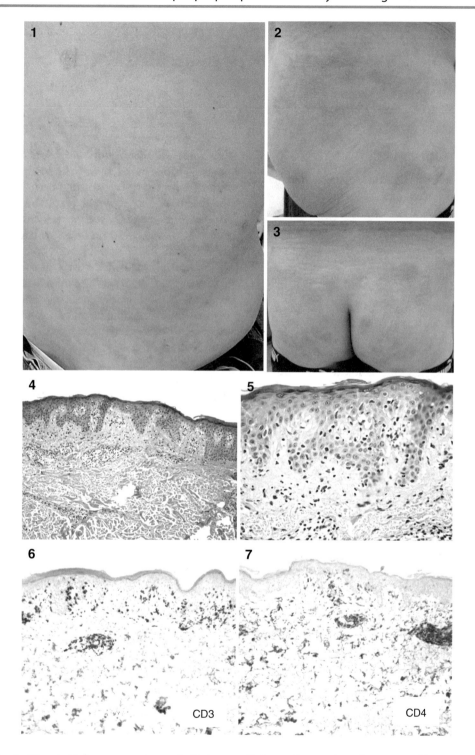

■ Fig. 1 The initial presentation of digitate patches on both flanks

■ Figs. 2 and 3 Six years, the classic patches of MF appeared on buttocks and the upper thighs in the bathing-trunk distribution

■ Fig. 4 Sparse lymphocytic infiltrate in the upper dermis, HE, ×2

■ Fig. 5 Marked lymphocytic epidermotropism, HE, ×10

■ Fig. 6 Atypical cells were positive for CD3

■ Fig. 7 Atypical cells were positive for CD4

Case 12. Extragenital Lichen Sclerosus et Atrophicans Mimicking Hypopigmented Mycosis Fungoides

V. Kazlouskaya, J. Ho, and O. E. Akilov

Age: 70   **Sex:** F

Clinical features: The Afro-American female was evaluated for flat, non-scaly, polygonal hypopigmented papules with cigarette paper-like wrinkled appearance on the chest, posterior neck, and bilateral dorsal hands present for a few months. Lesions were asymptomatic. The patient medical history was notorious for previously treated hepatitis C and a recent diagnosis of gastric cancer. A biopsy was taken and demonstrated a band-like infiltrate of lymphocytes underneath of the slightly homogenized upper dermis. Focal epidermotropism was noted and raised the possibility of mycosis fungoides. An infiltrate expressed CD3 and CD4 with a preserved expression of CD2, CD5, and CD7. T-cell rearrangement studies did not demonstrate monoclonality.

Diagnosis: Extragenital lichen sclerosus et atrophicans (LSetA) mimicking hypopigmented MF.

Follow-up: The rash did not progress over next 3 years.

Comment: LSetA and MF are two distinct conditions, but their clinical differential may be difficult at the early stages when the epidermal changes such as atrophy are not yet apparent. Moreover, histopathologically, there are cases of LSetA that have pronounced epidermotropism and simulate mycosis fungoides, and on some occasions, the distinction is not feasible. Homogenization and sclerosis of the upper dermis rather than thickened collagen bundles are more typical for LSetA but may be absent in the early stages of the disease. Moreover, a few cases with a classical presentation of LSetA were reported to harbor the monoclonal T-cell population contributing to the confusion. Isolated MF on the genital skin is extremely rare. While in this case, there was not genital involvement by LSetA, the distinction based on clinical presentation was possible to make. Different biopsies from the same patient may have different morphology in some cases displaying typical LSA features and, in other cases—the MF-like pictures. In those setting, clinical signs, distribution of the lesions, and clinical course are essential. Immunohistochemical findings and negative T-cell rearrangement, although not definitive, may be supportive in the distinction.

References

Citarella L, Massone C, Kerl H, Cerroni L. Lichen sclerosus with histopathologic features simulating early mycosis fungoides. Am J Dermatopathol. 2003;25:463–5.

Regauer S, Reich O, Beham-Schmid C. Monoclonal gamma-T-cell receptor rearrangement in vulvar lichen sclerosus and squamous cell carcinomas. Am J Pathol. 2002;160:1035–45.

Suchak R, Verdolini R, Robson A, Stefanato CM. Extragenital lichen sclerosus et atrophicus mimicking cutaneous T-cell lymphoma: report of a case. J Cutan Pathol. 2010;37:982–6.

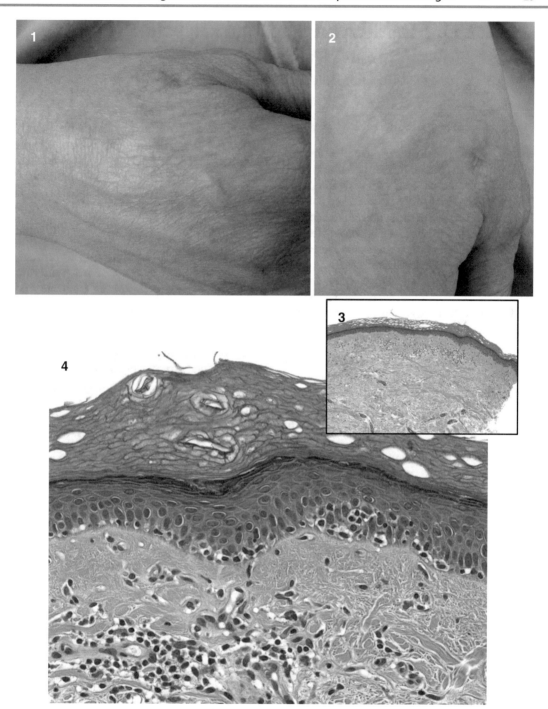

Case 13. T-Cell-Rich Angiomatoid Polypoid Pseudolymphoma (TRAPP) of the Skin

V. Kazlouskaya, J. Ho, and O. E. Akilov

Age: 21   **Sex:** F

Clinical features: The patient presented with a single lesion of concern on the left upper arm present for a few months, which was asymptomatic. The patient has a history of unspecified connective tissue disease with the symptoms suspicious for lupus (ANA 1:5120; low C3, chronic fatigue, and transient skin rashes) and is currently on hydroxychloroquine. The lesion was a 5 mm red papule surrounded by telangiectasias at the periphery. The biopsy showed the papillomatous epidermis with mild acanthosis overlying a superficial dermal lichenoid and interstitial infiltrate composed of a predominant population of small CD3+ T-cells admixed with a minor population of small CD20+ B-cells, and scattered histiocytes in a background of prominent vasculature. The lymphocytes had small hyperchromatic and mildly irregular nuclei. The infiltrate was predominantly dermal, with the only focal presence of lymphocytes in the epidermis. CD4 to CD8 ratio was within the normal range. Ki-67 proliferation index did not exceed 5% within the infiltrate.

Diagnosis: T-cell-rich angiomatoid polypoid pseudolymphoma (TRAPP).

Follow-up: Biopsy led to the total removal of the papule which did not recur during 1 year of follow-up.

Comment: TRAPP is a recently described T-cell pseudolymphoma clinically presenting as a single lesion with a benign course. It affects females more commonly and usually localized on the head and neck area, sometimes on the trunk. Although variable, more common histopathological features of TRAPP include the polypoid shape of the lesion, epidermal collarette, presence of Grenz zone, mildly atypical lymphocytes, and sometimes eosinophils in the infiltrate. Prominent vessels with slightly thickened walls or plumped cells are usually identified. TRAPP has overlapping features with acral pseudolymphomatous angiokeratoma of children (APACHE) and pretibial lymphoplasmacytic plaque (PLP). While some consider TRAPP and APACHE conditions of the same spectrum, the latter usually has mixed T-cell and B-cell infiltrate and presents with small solitary papules. PLP has numerous polyclonal plasma cells in the infiltrate and usually presents as a solitary plaque on young adults' lower extremities. Interestingly, patients with lupus erythematosus were described to have infiltrates, resembling lymphoproliferative disorders. Apart from more known presentations of lupus panniculitis and lymphocytic infiltration of Jessner, infiltrates resembling cutaneous CD4+ small-medium pleomorphic T-cell lymphoproliferative disorder, solitary T-cell pseudolymphoma, and low-grade cutaneous B-cell lymphomas were described as well.

References

Dayrit JF, Wang WL, Goh SG, Ramdial PK, Lazar AJ, Calonje E. T-cell-rich angiomatoid polypoid pseudo-lymphoma of the skin: a clinicopathologic study of 17 cases and a proposed nomenclature. J Cutan Pathol. 2011;38:475–82.

Fernandez-Flores A, Suarez Peñaranda JM, De Toro G, Alvarez Cuesta CC, Fernández-Figueras MT, Kempf W, Monteagudo C. Expression of peripheral node Addressins by Plasmacytic plaque of children, APACHE, TRAPP, and primary cutaneous angioplasmacellular hyperplasia. Appl Immunohistochem Mol Morphol. 2018;26:411–9.

Pereira A, Ferrara G, Calamaro P, Cota C, Massone C, Boggio F, Prieto-Torres L, Cerroni L. The histopathological spectrum of pseudolymphomatous infiltrates in cutaneous lupus erythematosus. Am J Dermatopathol. 2018;40:247–53.

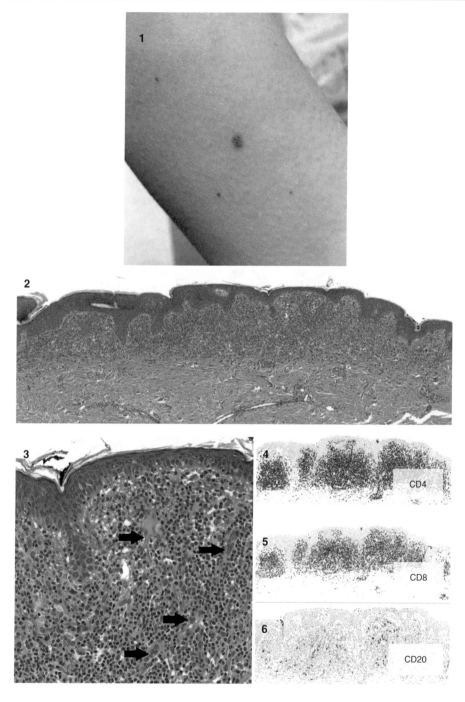

■ Fig. 1 Small slightly elevated papule on the left upper arm

■ Fig. 2 Band-like lymphocytic infiltrate in the upper dermis. HE, ×10

■ Fig. 3 High power demonstrating lymphoid infiltrate and prominent telangiectasias (arrows). HE, ×20

■ Fig. 4 Diffuse expression of CD4. ×10

■ Fig. 5 Numerous CD8 positive cell. ×10

■ Fig. 6 Few CD20 positive cells. ×10

Sezary Syndrome

While exfoliative or waxy erythroderma is a part of a triad for Sezary syndrome, it is not always present. Sezary syndrome in most of the case does not present diagnostic problems relying on the presence of more than 1000 clonal cells/mm3 in the peripheral blood. The difficulties arise with the choice of therapeutics in advanced leukemic cases when the cell number reaches more than 100,000 cells/mm3. The aberrant expression of CD30, CD26, and CD25 de novo is an indicator of poor prognosis.

Case 14. Pustular Sezary syndrome

O. E. AKILOV, J. HO, AND L. J. GESKIN

Age: 42   **Sex:** F

Clinical features: The patient with a 3-year history of lymphadenopathy, rash, and markedly atypical lymphocytosis in peripheral blood was diagnosed with Sezary syndrome, stage IVA2 (T4N3M0B2) 10 years ago. Flow cytometry demonstrated the atypical lymphocytes of memory type CD4+ CD45RO+ αβ T-cells, with weak CD25+ expression. Biopsy of inguinal lymph node revealed very prominent diffuse interfollicular expansion by a proliferation of small to intermediate size lymphoid cells with very irregular nuclear contours and occasional nucleoli. PCR analysis demonstrated a T-cell receptor γ-chain gene rearrangement. The patient had numerous therapies over the past several years, including ECP and interferon-α2a combination, denileukin diftitox, and gemcitabine without significant improvement. Six years prior, the patient was treated with ECP and bexarotene with a resolution of erythroderma and pruritus but relapsed 2 years later. Bexarotene was discontinued, and vorinostat (400 mg) was initiated in addition to monthly ECP treatments. A significant clinical response was noticed within 3 months, with nearly CR. The patient sustained clinical response for 6 months, at which point the dose had to be modified due to gastrointestinal side effects, and she experienced a relapse of her disease. The patient entered romidepsin (14 mg/m^2 on days 1, 8, and 15) clinical trial with erythroderma. The dose was increased by 25% to 17.5 mg/m^2 on Cycle 3 due to treatment benefit and minimal toxicity observed in this patient. Partial response (>50% of reduction) occurred by Cycle 6 steady regressing on average on 10% with each cycle. The patient received 16 cycles of this chemotherapy with LEBT during Cycle 10, 11, and 12 on resistant plaques. The romidepsin was discontinued due to disease progression, and pralatrexate was started. Unfortunately, her MF has progressed. The patient had an increase in the number of atypical lymphocytes in the peripheral blood (absolute lymphocyte count 30,000/mm^3). The patient developed multiple pustules on the background of palmoplantar keratoderma 1 week after 3 mg of alemtuzumab IV.

Diagnosis: Sezary syndrome, stage IVA2 (T4N3M0B2).

Follow-up: The lymphoma continued to progress in spite of treatment with alemtuzumab. Massive generalized lymphadenopathy was accompanied by the absolute lymphocyte count reaching the number of 60,000/mm^3 a month later in spite of alemtuzumab and pralatrexate combination. The patient developed staphylococcal bacterial otitis and eventually died of sepsis 2 months later after the presentation.

Comment: Pustular presentation of cutaneous T-cell lymphoma has been described before, although it remains to be an extremely rare phenomenon. It is considered to be an exaggerated Pautrier microabscesses reaching the visible size in a patient with advanced lymphoma.

Reference

Ackerman AB, Miller RC, Shapiro L. Pustular mycosis fungoides. Arch Dermatol. 1966;93:221–5.

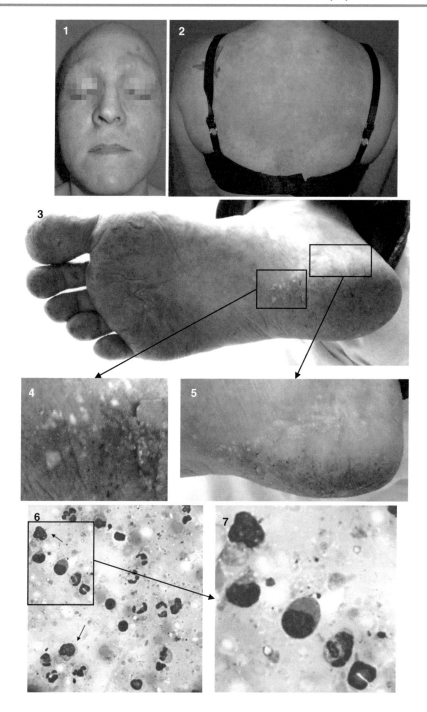

■ Fig. 1 Diffuse infiltration of the facial skin and alopecia totalis

■ Fig. 2 An infiltrative plaque on the upper back

■ Fig. 3 Callosities on the inflammatory background of the involved skin of the left sole surrounded by pustules

■ Fig. 4 1–2 mm well-defined pustules co-localized around callosities on the soles

■ Fig. 5 The medial surface of the left heal with pustules

■ Fig. 6 The content of the pustule demonstrates multiple atypical lymphocytes with neutrophils, Giemsa stain. ×100

■ Fig. 7 The high magnification of atypical lymphocytes in the content of a pustule. Giemsa stain, ×200

Case 15. De novo expression of CD26 on Sezary cells as an indicator of the disease progression in a patient with Sezary syndrome

S. Swerdlow and O. E. Akilov

Age: 67 **Sex:** F

Clinical features: The patient presented with a 4-year history of Sezary syndrome, stage IVA1 (T4N1M0B2) at diagnosis. She was treated with ECP, 15 cycles of romidepsin, and bexarotene 300 mg. She achieved CR with romidepsin infusions in the past. At the time of the first presented flow, she was enrolled in a clinical trial with an anti-CD47 compound when she received a single intralesional injection following by several weeks with pegylated interferon-alpha2a. Her disease eventually progressed, and the patient had restarted romidepsin. However, this time her leukemia was not controlled sufficiently with HDAC inhibitor only, requiring an intermittent subcutaneous injection of alemtuzumab and pegylated doxorubicin. The repeated flow, 4 months after treatment with romidepsin and alemtuzumab, demonstrated loss of CD4 expression on 51% of malignant cells and gain of CD26 expression on malignant lymphocytes (previously CD26 negative).

Diagnosis: Sezary syndrome, stage IVA2 (T4N3M0B2).

Follow-up: The patient developed massive lymphadenopathy (N3). The patient was planned to be enrolled in another clinical trial; however, her leukemic level reached the level of 120,000–350,000 cells/m^3, and the patient passed away.

Comment: This is the second report demonstrating that gaining CD26 expression by previously CD26 negative malignant cells as an indicator of unfavorable prognosis. The new expression in our patient coincides with the rapid leukemia progression of the previously controlled disease reaching unusually high count of >300,000 cells/mm^3 leading to fatal outcome.

Reference

Cedeno-Laurent F, Wysocka M, Obstfeld AE, et al. Gain of CD26 expression on the malignant T-cells in relapsed erythrodermic leukemic mycosis fungoides. J Cutan Pathol. 2017;44(5):462–6.

Fig. 1 Exfoliative erythroderma in a patient with Sezary syndrome

Fig. 2 Palmo-plantar keratoderma

Fig. 3 Multiple cutaneous erosion as a result of secondary skin infection in a patient with CD26+ Sezary cells

Fig. 4 Absolute lymphocyte and neutrophil count in response to various therapeutics between the first (CD26−) and the second (CD26+) flow cytometry results

Fig. 5 The first flow cytometry result demonstrating loss of CD7 and CD26 on Sezary cells. Published with kind permission of © Steven Swerdlow 2019. All Rights Reserved

Fig. 6 The second flow cytometry demonstrating gain of CD26 expression on Sezary cells. Note the loss of CD4 in 51% of cells. Published with kind permission of © Steven Swerdlow 2019. All Rights Reserved

Fig. 7 Multispectral imaging of the skin biopsy demonstrates the population of TOX+ Sezary cells with diminished expression of CD3 and CD4

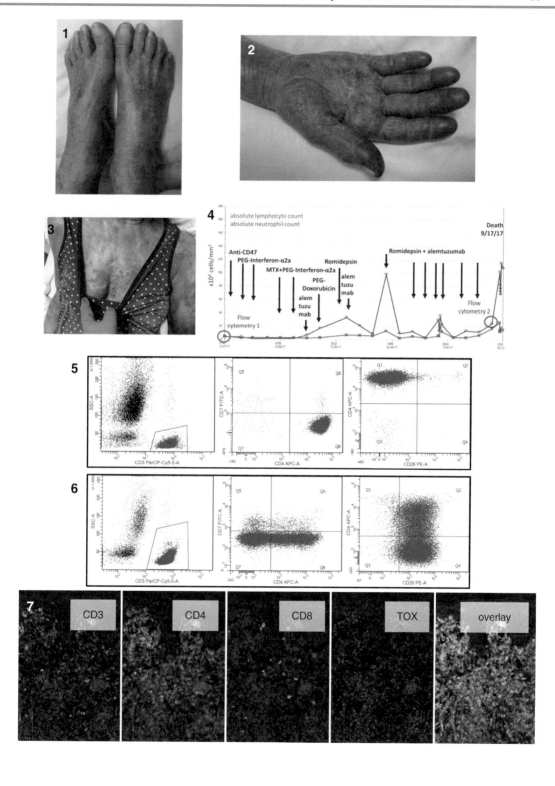

Case 16. Sezary syndrome presenting with papuloerythroderma of Ofuji and leonine facies

I. Litvinov

Age: 78   **Sex:** M

Clinical features: The patient presented with a 2-year history of Sezary syndrome, stage IVA1 (T4N1M0B2). His disease manifested by exfoliative erythroderma involving >90% body surface area, lymphadenopathy, painful and fissuring palmoplantar keratoderma with secondary hair loss and nail dystrophy. Notably, his face changed over time with plaques forming coarse features (leonine facies), while his erythroderma was notable for cobblestone appearance with a peculiar sparing of skin folds. The latter being consistent with the papuloerythroderma of Ofuji presentation of cutaneous lymphoma that was previously described. Human T-Cell Lymphotropic Virus-1 (HTLV-1) serology was negative. Multiple skin biopsies showed CD30+ expression on malignant lymphocytes. The patient had elevated lactate dehydrogenase level. Sezary cells accounted for ~75% of lymphocytes, CD4/CD8 T cell ratio was >10, with the positive clone on T-cell receptor (TCR) gene rearrangement studies.

Diagnosis: Sezary syndrome, stage IVA1 (T4N1M0B2).

Follow-up: The patient was suffering from intolerable pruritus requiring multimodal therapy and zopiclone to help him sleep. He also frequently presented to the hospital with the superinfection of the skin and pneumonia. In the past, he received methotrexate 12.5 mg orally weekly supplemented with folic acid and isotretinoin 40 mg daily. He attempted 6 months of treatment with phototherapy, which, unfortunately, failed to control his symptoms. Currently, his disease is stable on interferon-alpha 3 mln units 3 times a week, ECP, topical steroids, and N-acetyl cysteine 1200 mg twice daily.

Comments: This case highlights the importance of evaluating that papuloerythroderma of Ofuji or leonine facies could be the presenting features of CTCL.

References

Maher AM, Ward CE, Glassman S, Litvinov IV. The importance of excluding cutaneous T-cell lymphomas in patients with a working diagnosis of papuloerythroderma of ofuji: a case series. Case Rep Dermatol. 2018;10(1):46–54.

Oliveira A, Lobo I, Alves R, Lima M, Selores M. Sezary syndrome presenting with leonine facies and treated with low-dose subcutaneous alemtuzumab. Dermatol Online J. 2011;17(11):6.

■ **Fig. 1** Leonine facies in a patient with Sezary syndrome

■ **Fig. 2** Palmar keratoderma

■ **Fig. 3** "Deck Chair" sign is a characteristic of papuloerythroderma of Ofuji in a patient with Sezary syndrome

■ **Fig. 4** Islands of clear skin "in popleteal fossa" bilaterally in a patient with Sezary syndrome

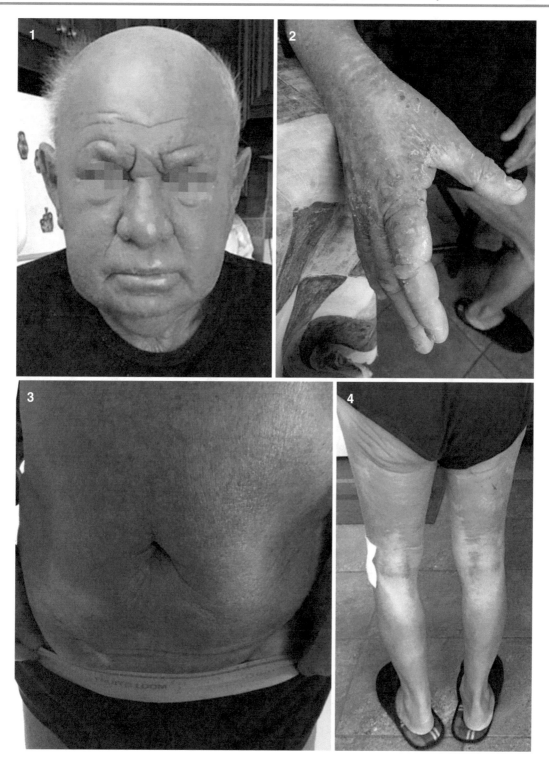

III CD30+ Lympho-proliferative Disorders

The number of reactive CD30+ infiltrates is disproportionally higher than cases of CD30+ lymphomas in the practice of dermatologists and oncologists. It should be a rule to exclude all benign conditions first in case of CD30+ cells' presence on biopsy since CD30 is not a marker of malignancy. Anaplastic large cell lymphoma is not a pediatric lymphoma. Paraphrasing a popular expression, the children's skin is not an adult skin in a small format. The cells appear to be more active and with ease acquire activation marker CD30 in cases of various arthropod assaults; the proliferative index is always high. Those morphologies without contest always look worrisome. Clinicopathologic correlation is crucial to avoid devastating treatments like in one of the cases below. CD30+ lymphoproliferative disorders present a spectrum of various conditions, and precise categorization sometimes remains to be difficult since there is some plasticity in clinical presentation as disease matures.

Case 17. Mycosis fungoides-like presentation of primary cutaneous anaplastic large cell lymphoma

A. Liu, S. Singh, J. Jedrych, J. Ho, and O. E. Akilov

Age: 82   **Sex:** F

Clinical features: The patient presented with erythematous patches and plaques with varying degrees of scaling and induration on the face, bilateral thighs, upper arms, and submammary spaces. A biopsy of one of the patches on her left medial thigh demonstrated an atypical T cell infiltrate with large cerebriform nuclei in the epidermis and dermal-epidermal junction concerning for MF. Repeat biopsy 3 months later showed numerous atypical, intraepidermal T cells with enlarged nuclei and irregular contours. Immuno-histochemical stains highlighted a monoclonal proliferation of atypical CD30+ CD5− CD7− T cells confined exceptionally to the epidermis. The patient was treated with ECP and topical steroids. One year later, the patient developed tumors on her left proximal arm and the right flank. A biopsy of the tumor demonstrated sheets of abnormal CD30+ lymphoid cells throughout the dermis with high Ki-67.

Diagnosis: Primary cutaneous anaplastic large cell lymphoma (pcALCL).

Follow-up: The patient was treated with two infusions of brentuximab vedotin with a significant decrease in tumor burden, despite severe complications of diarrhea, dehydration, and acute kidney injury. A residual tumor on the left thigh was treated with two cycles of localized electron beam therapy (LEBT), with a successful resolution. The patient's disease remains stable: she continues to use clobetasol ointment for any new patches.

Comment: pcALCL is a lymphoproliferative disorder that typically presents as a single or multiple nodules composed of CD30+ cells that form dermal-epidermal lymphoproliferative clusters or "sheets." MF, on the other hand, presents with pruritic patches and plaques, with tumors and erythroderma at the advanced stage. CD30+ cells could be observed in a subset of tumor patients with large cell transformation.

The differential diagnostics of tumor stage MF and pcACLC could be challenging in case of a limited history. Moreover, the appearance of pcALCL in patients with MF has been described previously, suggesting that along with LyP, those processes may present different phenotypical manifestations of the same T-cell clone. IRF4 translocation was recently proposed to be diagnostics for pcACLC being observed in 100% of those lymphomas, which could have been beneficial for our case. However, the presence of epidermotropic CD30+ lymphocytes at the initial presentation is suggestive of CD30+ LPD.

References

Cieza-Díaz DE, Prieto-Torres L, Rodríguez-Pinilla SM, et al. Mycosis fungoides associated with lesions in the spectrum of primary cutaneous CD30+ lymphoproliferative disorders: the same process or 3 coexisting lymphomas? Am J Dermatopathol. 2019;41(11):846–50.

Kiran T, Demirkesen C, Eker C, Kumusoglu H, Tuzuner N. The significance of MUM1/IRF4 protein expression and IRF4 translocation of CD30(+) cutaneous T-cell lymphoproliferative disorders: a study of 53 cases. Leuk Res. 2013;37(4):396–400.

Wu H, Telang GH, Lessin SR, Vonderheid EC. Mycosis fungoides with CD30-positive cells in the epidermis. Am J Dermatopathol. 2000;22(3):212–6.

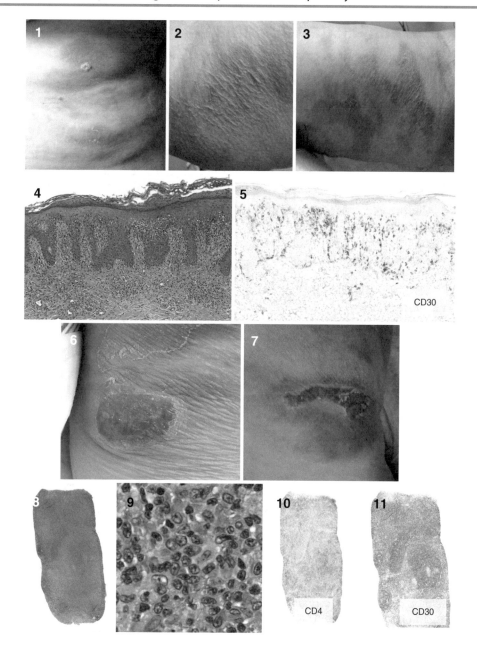

Figs. 1–3 Erythematous patches and thin plaques on the arm at time of the first biopsy

Fig. 4 Lichenoid infiltrate in a patch. HE, ×10

Fig. 5 CD30+ cells in the epidermis. ×40

Fig. 6 Large tumor on the right flank

Fig. 7 The resolution of the tumor after a single dose of brentuximab vedotin

Fig. 8 Sheets of atypical lymphocytes through the skin, HE, ×2

Fig. 9 Large atypical lymphocytes. HE, ×100

Fig. 10 CD4 positive cells. ×2

Fig. 11 CD30+ stain of sheets of abnormal lymphoid cells in the dermis from a biopsy of a nodule on the left arm

Case 18. Anaplastic lymphoma kinase-positive primary cutaneous anaplastic large cell lymphoma

R. C. MELCHERS, R. OTTEVANGER, AND K. D. QUINT

Age: 44   **Sex:** F

Clinical features: The patient presented with a solitary tumor on her left leg for the last 2 months. Microscopic examination of a biopsy revealed a diffuse dermal population of large anaplastic CD30-positive T-cells with combined nuclear and cytoplasmic anaplastic large cell lymphoma (ALK) expression. Additional investigations, including complete blood count, biochemical analysis, CT scan, and bone marrow biopsy, did not show visceral involvement.

Diagnosis: ALK-positive primary cutaneous anaplastic large cell lymphoma.

Follow-up: Radiotherapy (8 × 2.5 Gray) resulted in a complete remission. After a follow-up duration of 65 months, the patient was alive without disease.

Comment: PcALCL is an indolent cutaneous CD30+ T-cell lymphoma with no signs of extracutaneous localizations at the time of diagnosis. pcALCL is clinically characterized by single or localized, sometimes ulcerating tumors. Immunohistochemical characteristics are sheets of large anaplastic CD30+ cells. In contrast to systemic ALCL, the vast majority of pcALCL do not carry translocations of the *ALK* gene and do not express the ALK protein. Expression of ALK, therefore, strongly suggests a systemic ALK-positive ALCL with secondary cutaneous involvement. Nevertheless, our group observed that a small proportion of pcALCL cases (2%) harbor rearrangements involving the *ALK* gene. An immunohistochemical combined nuclear and cytoplasmic ALK staining suggests an underlying classical NPM-ALK translocation, while solely cytoplasmic expression suggests variant ALK fusion partners. ALK-positive and negative pcALCL have a comparable, excellent prognosis and should be treated with radiotherapy as the first treatment option.

References

Benharroch D, Meguerian-Bedoyan Z, Lamant L, et al. ALK-positive lymphoma: a single disease with a broad spectrum of morphology. Blood. 1998;91:2076–84.

Geller S, Canavan TN, Pulitzer M, et al. ALK-positive primary cutaneous anaplastic large cell lymphoma: a case report and review of the literature. Int J Dermatol. 2018;57:515–20.

Melchers RC, Willemze R, van de Loo M, et al. Clinical, histological and molecular characteristics of anaplastic lymphoma kinase-positive primary cutaneous anaplastic large cell lymphoma. Am J Surg Pathol. 2020;44(6):776–81.

Oschlies I, Lisfeld J, Lamant L, et al. ALK-positive anaplastic large cell lymphoma limited to the skin: clinical, histopathological and molecular analysis of 6 pediatric cases. A report from the ALCL99 study. Haematologica. 2013;98:50–6.

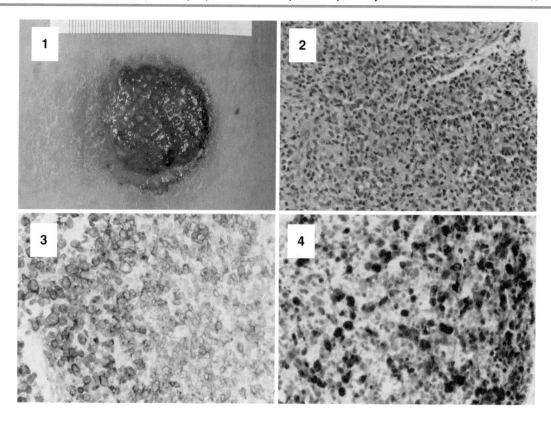

◾ Fig. 1 Single ulcerated tumor of 5 × 5 cm on the leg

◾ Fig. 2 Diffuse dermal infiltrate with large anaplastic cells

◾ Fig. 3 CD30 expression

◾ Fig. 4 ALK expression in the nucleus and cytoplasm

Case 19. Successful treatment of primary cutaneous anaplastic large cell lymphoma on the penile shaft with brentuximab vedotin and allogenic stem cell transplant

J. Yoo, A. Stevens, S. Chaganti, and J. Scarisbrick

Age: 48   **Sex:** M

Clinical features: The patient presented with 4-year history of widespread patches and plaques and 2 months history of penile tumor. The skin biopsy diffuse lymphocytic infiltrates positive for CD30 and CD45 while being negative for ALK-1. The initial staging workup demonstrated the absence of systemic involvement confirming the diagnosis of primary cutaneous anaplastic large cell lymphoma (pcALCL). Following 2 cycles of CHOP and radiotherapy (30 Gy in 15 fractions for penile tumor and 20 Gy in five fractions for left calf tumor), complete remission was achieved. The patient had skin-limited relapses on the right pubic area 4 months after CR and the left fifth finger 13 months after CR, which resulted in spontaneous resolution. A month later, he developed a large swelling on the left side of the pelvis. PET/CT followed by core needle lymph node biopsy confirmed secondary involvement of left iliac nodes with pcALCL. Brentuximab vedotin (BV) was initiated and complete remission was achieved at cycle 4 which was continued further until cycle 8. Once complete remission was achieved, total lymphoid irradiation and anti-thymocyte globulin (TLI/ATG)-conditioned sex-matched sibling allogeneic hematopoietic stem cell transplantation was performed. The patient successfully was treated with three donor leukocyte infusion for low chimerism and remains in complete remission 5 years after the transplant.

Diagnosis: pcALCL with a relapse into a regional lymph node, Ann Arbor, stage I.

Comments: pcALCL is a rare CD30+ lymphoproliferative disorder with excellent prognosis (10-year disease-specific survival = 96%) despite frequent cutaneous relapses. The 5-year cumulative risk of systemic progression is 14% most commonly within the first 2 years (80%) and all within 4 years. Chemotherapy with consideration of allo-HSCT if eligible has been considered as the first-line treatment for systemic relapse in the past although there is a lack of large-scale data to support this. BV (anti-CD30 monoclonal antibody conjugated to vedotin) is now an important treatment option for patients with CD30+ pcALCL and it has been approved by the Food and Drug Administration and European Commissions in 2017. An international, open-label, randomised, phase 3, multicentre trial (ALCANZA) comparing BV against physician's choice (oral methotrexate or bexarotene) in patients with CD30-positive mycosis fungoides or pcALCL, showed the objective response rate lasting at least 4 months (ORR4) of 56.3% with BV versus 12.5% with physician's choice. Peripheral neuropathy was common side effects with BV (67%). BV has potential role providing an alternative to chemotherapy to bridge to transplant. Our case demonstrates successful treatment of pcALCL with the regional lymph node involvement with allo-HSCT.

References

Bekkenk MW, Geelen FA, van Voorst Vader PC, et al. Primary and secondary cutaneous CD30(+) lymphoproliferative disorders: a report from the Dutch Cutaneous Lymphoma Group on the long-term follow-up data of 219 patients and guidelines for diagnosis and treatment. Blood. 2000;95:3653–61.

Hapgood G, Pickles T, Sehn LH, et al. Outcome of primary cutaneous anaplastic large cell lymphoma: a 20-year British Columbia Cancer Agency experience. Br J Haematol. 2017;176:234–40.

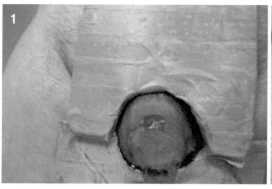

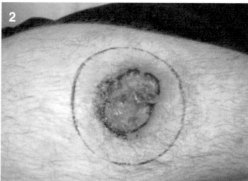

Pre-treatment PET-CT 07.06.2014 showing an FDG avid left pelvic lymph node mass

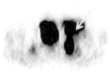 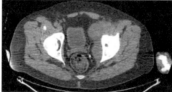 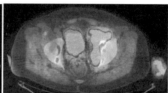

Post-treatment PET-CT 16.12.2014 showing a complete response.

 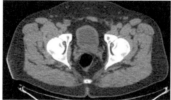 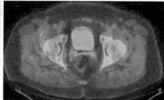

■ Fig. 1 Ulcerated nodule on the penile shaft
■ Fig. 2 Ulcerated nodule on the left calf
■ Fig. 3 PET/CT at the time of systemic progression

■ Fig. 4 PET/CT after 8 cycles of brentuximab vedotin

Case 20. Lymphomatoid papulosis type D in a child with CD8+ hypopigmented mycosis fungoides

I. E. Belousova and W. Kempf

Age: 9   **Sex:** M

Clinical features: The patient with a 6.5-year history of recurrent self-resolved necrotic papulo-nodules started noticing small erythematous patches on the trunk 5.5 years after papules' appearance. Both types of lesions left post-inflammatory hypopigmentation. No lymph-adenopathy on the physical exam. Peripheral blood counts were within normal limits. The biopsy was taken from the patch on the hand and the papule on the trunk. The papule's histology showed a V-shaped epidermotropic infiltrate of small CD3+ CD8+ lymphocytes with an admixture of large atypical, mostly intraepidermal lymphoid cells with a CD3+ CD4− CD8+ CD30+ phenotype. The biopsy from the patch showed a superficial epidermotropic infiltrate of small- to medium-sized cerebriform lymphocytes with a CD2dim CD3+ CD4− CD5dim CD8+ CD30− immunophenotype. The T-cell receptor gene rearrangement analysis revealed a dominant clone identical in both specimens.

Diagnosis: CD8+ hypopigmented mycosis fungoides and CD8+ lymphomatoid papulosis (LyP, type D or CD8+ epidermotropic) in a child.

Follow-up: The patient received three courses of NB UVB over 5 years, which resulted in complete resolution of the patches and reduced papules number.

Comment: Cutaneous lymphomas usually affect the elderly but may sometimes present as early as during the first decade. MF and LyP are the two most common lymphomas in children. In contrast to the classic Alibert-Bazin type of MF typically seen in adults, hypopigmented MF appears to be the most prevalent form in pediatric patients. The CD8+ phenotype seems to be more frequent in children and, in fact, also was found to be in our patient. The clinical presentation of LyP in children is similar to that seen in adults. Juvenile-onset MF may be associated with LyP in up to 18%.

In our case, the challenging diagnostic question is whether all the papular lesions can be regarded as LyP or should be considered a papular MF. The presence of the same clone does not exclude the possibility of two diagnoses. In our case, the papules were enriched by epidermotropic CD30+ large atypical cells arguing in favor of a separate lymphoproliferative disease. We considered PLEVA; however, morphologically, those papules without a collarette-like scale were more consistent with LyP.

References

Ferenczi K, Makkar HS. Cutaneous lymphoma: kids are not just little people. Clin Dermatol. 2016;34(6):749–59.

Kempf W, Kazakov DV, Palmedo G, Fraitag SL, Kutzner H. Pityriasis lichenoides et varioliformis acuta with numerous CD30(+) cells: a variant mimicking lymphomatoid papulosis and other cutaneous lymphomas. A clinicopathologic, immunohistochemical, and molecular biological study of 13 cases. Am J Surg Pathol. 2012;36(7):1021–9.

Kempf W, Kazakov DV, Belousova IE, Mitteldorf C, Kerl K. Paediatric cutaneous lymphomas: a review and comparison with adult counterparts. J Eur Acad Dermatol Venereol. 2015;29(9):1696–709.

Wieser I, Wohlmuth C, Nunez CA, Duvic M. Lymphomatoid papulosis in children and adolescents: a systematic review. Am J Clin Dermatol. 2016;17(4):319–27.

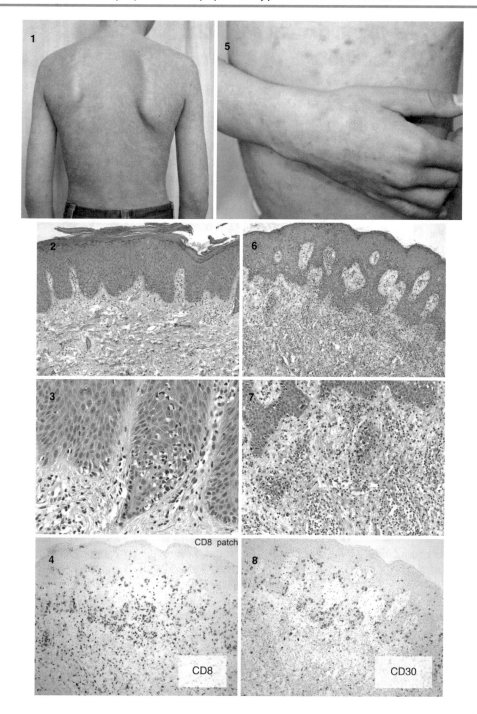

■ Fig. 1 Hypopigmented MF patches on the trunk

■ Figs. 2 and 3 Superficial epidermotropic infiltrate of small- to medium-sized cerebriform lymphocytes forming Pautrier's microabscess

■ Fig. 4 CD8 expression on the intraepidermal atypical lymphocytes

■ Fig. 5 Red, hemorrhagic, and necrotic papules on the trunk

■ Figs. 6 and 7 Epidermotropic infiltrate of small and large atypical lymphoid cells

■ Fig. 8 CD30 expression on the intraepidermal atypical lymphocytes

Case 21. Lymphomatoid papulosis and autoimmunity

Helen Ma and Ahmed Sawas

Age: 63 **Sex:** F

Clinical features: A patient with history of celiac disease developed erythematous papules in the left axilla (Fig. 1). A punch biopsy was performed. Immunohistochemistry was positive for CD3, CD4, CD5, CD7 (partial loss), CD8, and CD30 (10–15%). Pathology was concerning for mycosis fungoides (MF) with large cell transformation. Peripheral blood flow cytometry revealed no blood involvement. Positron emission tomography and computed tomography (PET/CT) revealed a 3.2 × 2.7cm ground glass opacity in the right upper lobe. Surgical lobectomy showed stage 1 lung adenocarcinoma. For the apparent "transformed MF" in the left axilla, the patient underwent radiation therapy. Afterwards, she developed new lesions on her arms, abdomen, and lower extremities. Biopsy of right axillary lesion showed a dense lymphoid infiltrate in upper dermis with epidermotropism. The atypical cells were medium sized and positive for CD3, CD8, CD30 (partial), CD25 (partial) with Ki67 40–50%. The patient started brentuximab vedotin, but did not notice any improvment in her lesions. The repeat biopsy showed two lymphoid T-cell populations with varying in expression of CD4, CD8, CD30, and Ki67 (Fig. 2). The patient presented for consultation.

Diagnosis: Lymphomatoid papulosis.

Follow-up: The patient was treated with topical clobetasol 0.05% resulting in a resolution of lesions without recurrence. About 6 months later, she developed proximal muscle weakness with difficulty holding up her head. Head CT and lumbar puncture were unrevealing, but Magnetic resonance imaging (MRI) of the spine showed paraspinal edema from C4 to T3. Laboratory analysis showed antibodies against dsDNA and rheumatoid factor with an elevated creatine kinase (CK). Biopsy of muscle showed necrotic/regenerating and atrophic fibers in perifascicular pattern, consistent with dermatomyositis. T-cell receptor gene rearrangement was polyclonal by PCR. Electromyography demonistrated chronic myopathic changes without active denervation. PET/CT revealed cutaneous infiltrative changes with slight Fluorodeoxyglucose uptake (SUV 2.2) in the left anterior upper thigh and dorsal to the L3 vertebral body and spinal accessory muscle (SUV 3.7) (Fig. 3). She improved on prednisone (40mg daily) and methotrexate 20 mg weekly. With treatment, the muscle weakness improved, and she no longer was wheelchair bound.

Comments: Chronic inflammation and antigen stimulation seen in autoimmune disease (AID) have been associated with the development of lymphoma with reported odds ratio (OR) of 2.6; 95% CI = 1.7–4.07 but generally the AID precedes the lymphoma diagnosis. In dermatomyositis, antibodies activate compliment and membrane attack complexes deposit endothelial cells and capillaries that lead to ischemia. There is also possible "paraneoplastic" association because AID improved after treatment of lymphoma though this was not the case in our patient. There are also case reports of dermatomyositis that preceded a T-cell lymphoma diagnosis.

References

Mellemkjaer L, et al. Autoimmune disease in individuals and close family members and susceptibility to non-Hodgkin's lymphoma. Arthritis Rheum. 2008;58(3):657–66.

Pasquet F, et al. [Autoimmune diseases and cancers. Part I: cancers complicating autoimmune diseases and their treatment]. Rev Med Interne. 2014;35(5):310–6.

Reed AM, Ytterberg SR. Genetic and environmental risk factors for idiopathic inflammatory myopathies. Rheum Dis Clin N Am. 2002;28(4):891–916.

Stubgen JP. Inflammatory myopathies and lymphoma. J Neurol Sci. 2016;369:377–89.

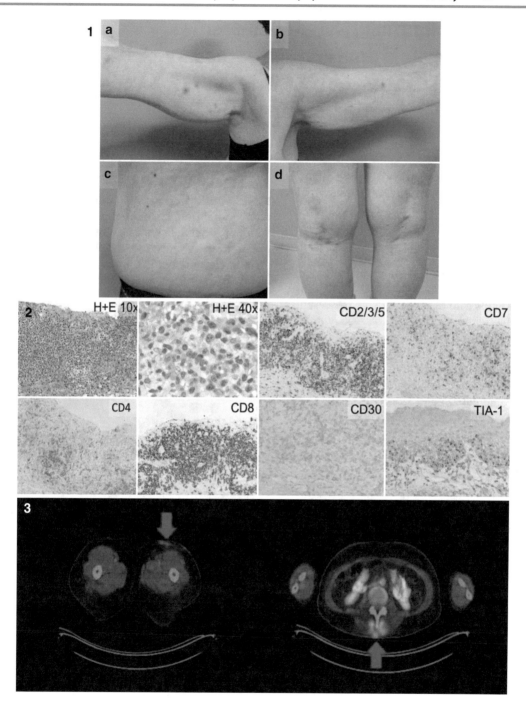

Fig. 1 Erythematous papules on (a) ventral aspect of right arm and axilla, (b) ventral aspect of left arm and axilla, (c) abdomen, and (d) bilateral popliteal fossae

Fig. 2 Two population of atypical cells: (1) one within the superficial component positive for CD2, CD3, CD8, CD30 (>25%), CD4 (weak), CD5 (weak), and Ki67 60–70%; and (2) one within the subjacent component positive for CD2, CD3, CD4, CD8 (subset), CD5 (strong), and CD30 (<25%), and Ki67 10–20%

Fig. 3 PET/CT with inflammatory changes (arrows) without evidence of FDG-avid disease in lymph nodes, skin, or other masses

Case 22. Infusion-related CD30-positive lymphomatoid drug eruption secondary to melphalan

M. Matsumoto, J. Ho, and O. E. Akilov

Age: 66   **Sex:** M

Clinical features: A patient with mantle cell lymphoma developed pruritic, indurated papules on his right chest and shoulder surrounding his port site on day 2 of carmustine, etoposide, cytarabine, melphalan (BEAM) induction prior to autologous stem cell transplant. Skin histology demonstrated spongiotic dermatitis with dyskeratosis, focal basal vacuolar change, eosinophils with dense superficial perivascular and interstitial atypical and enlarged lymphoid cells, positive for CD4 and CD30 and negative for CD20, Cyclin D1, ALK1. Ki-67 stain highlighted 40% of enlarged lymphoid cells. Physical examination, complete blood count and differential, and comprehensive metabolic panel at time of onset were otherwise unremarkable.

Diagnosis: Infusion-related CD30+ lymphomatoid drug eruption secondary to melphalan.

Follow-up: Drug eruption was not responsive to treatment with two doses of systemic methylprednisolone and topical triamcinolone ointment. Patient underwent successful autologous stem cell transplant with improvement noted in rash 2 weeks following last dose of melphalan.

Comment: CD30+ lymphomatoid drug eruptions generally present as erythematous papulonodules, most commonly on the trunk or extremities, 1 week to months after drug exposure. Reported causative agents include statins, antihypertensives, immunomodulators, antibiotics, chemotherapy agents, and antidepressants. Three cases of CD30+ lymphoproliferative disorders developing post-melphalan treatment have been reported. On histology, CD30+ lymphomatoid drug eruptions present with eosinophils, papillary dermal edema, spongiosis, interface dermatitis, and superficial perivascular infiltrates of large, atypical CD4+ CD30+ polyclonal lymphoid cells without cytotoxic phenotype.

References

Chen YC, Wu YH. Linear folliculotropic CD30-positie lymphomatoid drug reaction. Am J Dermatopathol. 2017;39(5):e62–5.

Gill K, Ariyan C, Wang X, Brady MS, Pulitzer M. CD30-positive lymphoproliferative disorders arising after regional therapy for recurrent melanoma: a report of two cases and analysis of CD30 expression. J Surg Oncol. 2014;110(3):258–64.

Magro CM, Olson LC, Nguyen GH, de Feraudy SM. CD30 positive lymphomatoid angiocentric drug reactions: characterization of a series of 20 cases. Am J Dermatopathol. 2017;39(7):508–17.

Qian YW, Siegel D, Bhattacharyya P. Multiple skin lesions in a patient with multiple myeloma. CD30-positive cutaneous large cell lymphoproliferative disorder. Arch Pathol Lab Med. 2006;130:e41–3.

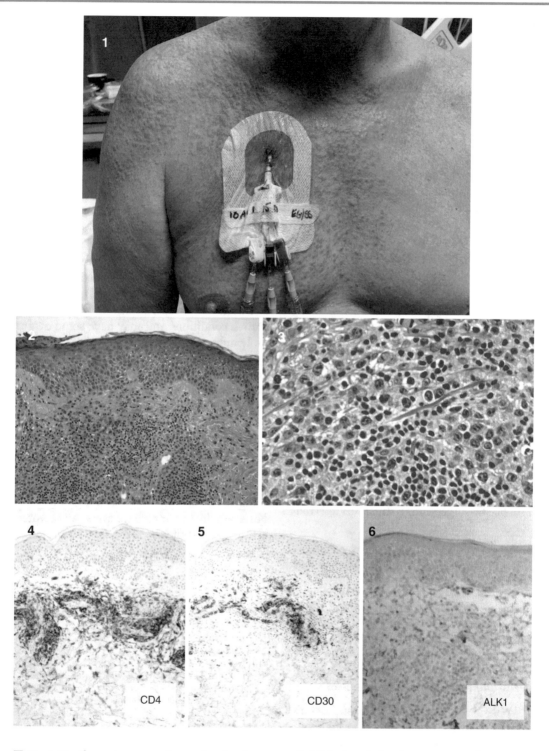

■ Fig. 1 Erythematous papules coalescing into plaques over R chest and shoulder surrounding port

■ Figs. 2 and 3 Dense perivascular infiltrate of large, atypical cells with spongiosis, dyskeratosis, eosinophils, and focal interface change.

Published with kind permission of © Jonhan Ho 2019. All Rights Reserved

■ Figs. 4–6 Large cells expressed CD4 and CD30. ALK1 is negative. Published with kind permission of © Jonhan Ho 2019. All Rights Reserved

Case 23. Arthropod reaction with CD30 positive infiltrate and ulceration mimicking CD30 lymphoproliferative disorder

V. Kazlouskaya, J. Ho, and O. E. Akilov

Age: 10 years **Sex:** M

Clinical features: Patient presented with erythematous papular lesions on the trunk with minimal scale and larger ulcerated lesion on the cheek of few months of duration. Patient was otherwise healthy. Tissue cultures did not demonstrate microorganisms. Biopsy of the ulcerated lesion was performed and showed a necrotic tissue with underlying inflammatory infiltrate. Infiltrate had mixed cells including lymphocytes, neutrophils, and numerous eosinophils. A cluster of atypical lymphocytes was noted at the edge of the biopsy with atypical cells diffusely expressing CD30. Lymphocytes were also stained for CD4, with only few CD20 positive cells and diminished expression of CD5, CD7, and CD8. PD-1 and CXCL13 were negative, as well as infectious stains. Pediatric hematologist was concerned of CD30+ lymphoma. The infectious disease doctor suggested to perform deep excisional biopsy and recommended to schedule an excision with plastic surgery. The patient was referred to our center for a second opinion.

Diagnosis: Arthropod reaction with CD30 positive infiltrate and ulceration mimicking CD30 lymphoproliferative condition.

Follow-up: We ruled lymphoma. Bone marrow biopsy was not necessary as well as stem cell transplant. We recommended to avoid deep excision biopsy on the face. Lesions have resolved on its own and the boy is in good health and free from lesions for 4 years.

Comment: Although diffuse infiltrates of CD30 positive cells are seen in lymphoproliferative disorders such as lymphomatous papulosis and anaplastic large cell lymphoma, clusters of lymphocytes expressing CD30 marker may be seen in numerous non-neoplastic conditions such as infections (varicella zoster, molluscum contagiosum, syphilis, Borrelia, etc.), drug reactions, hidradenitis, pernio among others. Sometimes these clusters are non-specific and are occasionally discovered in the biopsies on re-excisions of other non-related conditions such as epidermal cysts or neoplasms. Scabies infiltrates are known to mimic lymphoproliferative conditions and may have some degree of lymphocytic atypia, but similar reactions were described after tick or spider bites, and arthropod assaults. These lesions may persist long after the infestation and cause a diagnostic dilemma. In case of spider bite, the concentration of CD30 positive cells was reported to be up to 25% per power field. Long-term follow-up and detailed clinical information is essential to establish the correct diagnosis and avoid medical crisis such as unnecessary stem cell transplantation after conditioning regimens. For example, in our case we eventually favored arthropod assault with secondary ulceration.

References

Ccepeda LT, Pieretti M, Chapman SF, Horenstein MG. CD30-positive atypical lymphoid cells in common non-neoplastic cutaneous infiltrates rich in neutrophils and eosinophils. Am J Surg Pathol. 2003;27:912–8.

Hwong H, Jones D, Prieto VG, Schulz C, Duvic M. Persistent atypical lymphocytic hyperplasia following tick bite in a child: report of a case and review of the literature. Pediatr Dermatol. 2001;18:481–4.

Werner B, Massone C, Kerl H, Cerroni L. Large CD30-positive cells in benign, atypical lymphoid infiltrates of the skin. J Cutan Pathol. 2008;35:1100–7.

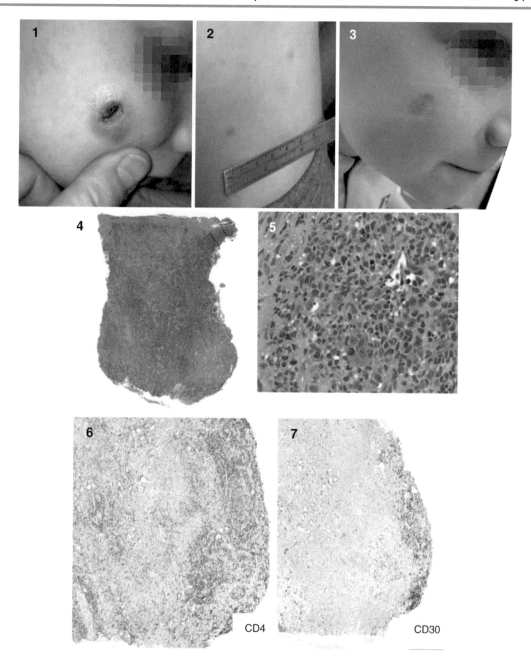

Fig. 1 Larger ulcerated lesion on the left cheek

Fig. 2 Erythematous urticarial papules on the trunk with minimal scale

Fig. 3 Resolution of the lesion with no treatment

Fig. 4 Scanning magnification demonstrating an ulcer with tissue necrosis and underlying lymphocytic infiltrate

Fig. 5 Higher magnification shows mixed infiltrate with numerous eosinophils and atypical medium sized lymphocytes with irregular nuclei and hyperchromasia

Fig. 6 Infiltrate is diffusely expressing CD4

Fig. 7 Cluster of CD30 positive cells that correspond to the area of atypical lymphocytes

IV Extranodal NK/T-Cell Lymphoma

NK/T-cell lymphomas are extremely rare lymphomas in the western world. The population of CD3+CD56+ NK/T-cells that seems to be the progenitor cells for those types of lymphomas is not homogeneous, which may explain the reason for polymorphic presentation. Several functionally distinct NK/T-cell subsets diverge after their development in the thymus. Organ-specific antigen-presenting cells may modulate NK/T-cell function and post-thymic development. The organs with the highest content of NK/T cells are tonsils, lymph nodes, spleen, skin, testis, and stomach. Not surprisingly, those are the places of the most frequent localization of NK/T-cell lymphoma. The Waldeyer's tonsillar ring is involved most commonly. The patient sometimes may present with a single cutaneous nodule, but the asymptomatic nasal involvement could be detected on PET/CT frequently, still placing the patient into "the nasal" category. Extranasal presentation comprises around 20% of all cases and most likely arises from the dermal NK/T cells in contrast to tonsillar NK/T cells in "the nasal" cases. Unusual cases of such rare cancer are characterized by the unusual expression of non-NK/T-cell markers and rare morphologic presentations. The aberrant expression of $\gamma\delta$ TCR on EBV+ CD56+ cells is still a matter of debate of appropriate classificational categorization. Despite semantics, the prognosis is universally gravid.

Case 24. Extranodal NK/T-Cell lymphoma, nasal type

K. Severson, A. Rosenthal, D. DiCaudo, and A. Mangold

Age: 79   **Sex:** M

Clinical features: Large, fungating tumors developed over 6 weeks in a patient with chronic lymphocytic leukemia (CLL) on ibrutinib. Physical exam demonstrated 15 cm masses along his posterior neck and left axilla. Flow cytometry on the initial skin biopsy showed an aberrant cell population positive for CD2, CD4, HLA-DR, partial cytoplasmic CD3 and diminished CD45 with negative CD56. Additional biopsies showed deep dermal infiltrate of atypical cells with frequent mitoses, angiocentricity, and focal angiodestruction. Cells were positive for CD3, CD4, CD5, CD43, weak CD56 and were negative for CD8, TIA-1, and granzyme B. EBV (Epstein-Barr virus) was positive by in situ hybridization. No atypical populations involved the peripheral blood or bone marrow. PET/CT can demonstrate involvement of the laryngo-nasal area, right subclavicular and left axillary lymph nodes. Labs revealed elevated LDH of 505 U/L and plasma EBV PCR of 48,700 IU/mL. Ibrutinib was stopped.

Diagnosis: Extranodal NK T-cell lymphoma, nasal type (ENKTCL).

Follow-up: DDGP (Dexamethasone, Cisplatin, Gemcitabine, Peg-Asparaginase) was initiated with approximately 90% reduction of tumors after one cycle.

Comment: ENKTCL is a rare, aggressive frequently highly associated with EBV. While the most commonly involved sites include the nose/sinus with presenting symptoms of obstruction or epistaxis, extranodal skin sites present with necrosis from angiodestruction. ENKTCL is often CD56 (75%), CD2, cytoplasmic CD3 epsilon, CD43, CD45RO and cytotoxic marker positive. Cases which are CD3(+), CD56(−) are considered ENKTCL if EBV and cytotoxic markers are positive. Non-classical or EBV(−) cases may be best regarded as peripheral T-cell lymphomas not otherwise specified. DDGP may offer better response rates with less toxicity compared to SMILE (dexamethasone, methotrexate, ifosfamide, L-asparaginase, and etoposide).

References

Allen P, Lechowicz MJ. Management of NK/T-cell lymphoma, nasal type. J Oncol Pract. 2019;15:513–20.

Au W-Y, Weisenburger DD, et al. Clinical differences between nasal and extranasal natural killer/T-cell lymphoma: a study of 136 cases from the International Peripheral T-Cell Lymphoma Project. Blood. 2009;113(17):3931–7.

Li X, Cui Y, et al. DDGP versus SMILE in newly diagnosed advanced natural killer/T-cell lymphoma: a randomized controlled, multicenter, open-label study in China. Clin Cancer Res. 2016;22(21):5223–8.

Vainder C, Ho J, et al. CD56− extranodal natural killer (NK)/T-cell lymphoma, nasal type presenting as skin ulcers in a white man. JAAD Case Rep. 2016;2(5):390–6.

Fig. 1 Posterior neck ulcerative tumor, pre- (**a**) and post-treatment (**b**). Published with kind permission of © From Mayo Foundation for Medical Education and Research. All rights reserved

Fig. 2 Whole body PET/CT. Published with kind permission of © From Mayo Foundation for Medical Education and Research. All rights reserved

Fig. 3 Angiodestructive infiltrate involving medium-sized vessel, HE 200× (**a**); Angiotropic infiltrate of pleomorphic large cells with zones of necrosis, HE 200× (**b**); CD3 focal positivity, 200× (**c**); CD4 positive, 200× (**d**); CD56 rare cells with weak positivity, 400× (**e**); EBER diffusely positive, 200× (**f**). Published with kind permission of © From Mayo Foundation for Medical Education and Research. All rights reserved

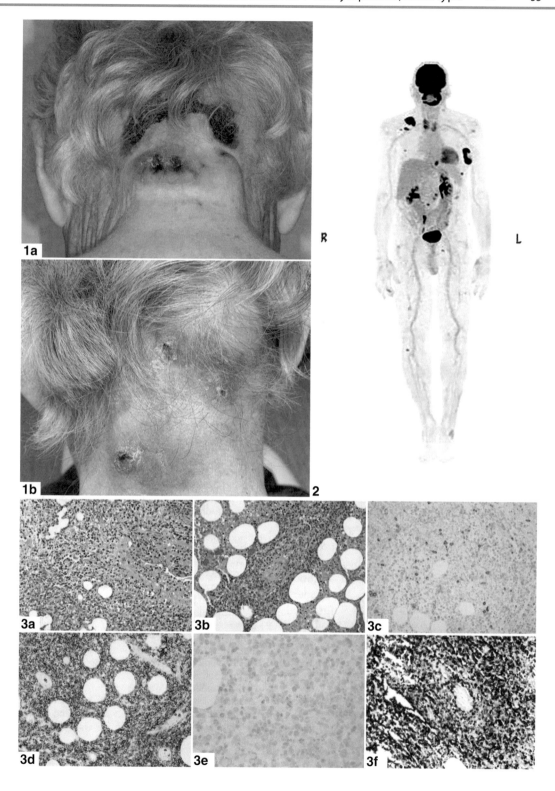

Case 25. EBV-associated extranodal NK/T-Cell lymphoma with γ/δ TCR expression presented as aphthous stomatitis

F. Dimitriou, M. -C. Brüggen, and E. Guenova

Age: 87 **Sex:** F

Clinical features: The patient presented with necrotizing gingivitis with a 2-month history of painful oral aphthous stomatitis and gingival bleeding. A local treatment with disinfecting rinsing agents was initiated, without effect. Clinical examination showed a solitary grayish, infiltrated and ulcerated plaque on the upper palate and multiple mucosal small aphthous ulcerations. A mucosal biopsy showed a CD3+/CD2+, cytotoxic (perforin+/granzyme B+/TIA1–/TdT–), highly proliferative infiltrate. The cells exhibited partial (30%) co-expression of CD30 and CD56, but were completely negative for CD4, CD8, CD5, and CD7. TCRγ/δ gamma (but not TCR-β-F1) and EBV-encoded small nuclear RNA (EBER) was found on/in the tumor cells.

Diagnosis: EBV-associated ENKTL nasal type with γ/δ TCR expression.

Follow-up: Positron emission tomography-computed tomography (PET-CT) showed multiple metabolically active focuses and bone lesions. Due to the aberrant CD30 expression, a systemic treatment with brentuximab-vedotin, an anti-CD30 monoclonal antibody drug, was proposed. However, the patient refused any treatment intervention and died due to disease progression and sepsis 64 days after the diagnosis.

Comment: Mature T- and NK-cell malignancies are rare. The 2008 WHO classification, revised in 2016, recognizes extranodal NK/T-cell lymphoma (ENKTL) as one of the prototypes of virally associated Epstein–Barr virus (EBV)-positive T-cell or NK-cell lymphoma. ENKTL, nasal type affects adult individuals, predominantly males and is more frequent in Asia, Mexico, and South America. The prototypic immunophenotype of ENKTL is CD2+CD56+. Surface CD3 and other common T-cell antigens (CD4, CD8, CD5) are usually negative with positivity for cytoplasmic CD3ε. Some tumors express α/β-T-cell receptor (α/β-TCR). γ/δ TCR expression has rarely been reported and molecular analysis only rarely detects a monoclonal rearrangement of the TCR gene. Characteristically, EBV can be detected in almost all cases of ENKTL. This case emphasizes the importance of a rapid histological examination and treatment of refractory oral lesions.

References

Bruggen MC, Kerl K, Haralambieva E, Schanz U, Chang YT, Ignatova D, et al. Aggressive rare T-cell lymphomas with manifestation in the skin: a monocentric cross-sectional case study. Acta Derm Venereol. 2018;98(9):835–41.

Kato S, Asano N, Miyata-Takata T, Takata K, Elsayed AA, Satou A, et al. T-cell receptor (TCR) phenotype of nodal Epstein-Barr virus (EBV)-positive cytotoxic T-cell lymphoma (CTL): a clinicopathologic study of 39 cases. Am J Surg Pathol. 2015;39(4):462–71.

Pongpruttipan T, Sukpanichnant S, Assanasen T, Wannakrairot P, Boonsakan P, Kanoksil W, et al. Extranodal NK/T-cell lymphoma, nasal type, includes cases of natural killer cell and alphabeta, and alphabeta/gammadelta T-cell origin: a comprehensive clinicopathologic and phenotypic study. Am J Surg Pathol. 2012;36(4):481–99.

Vose J, Armitage J, Weisenburger D, International TCLP. International peripheral T-cell natural killer/T-cell lymphoma study: pathology findings and clinical outcomes. J Clin Oncol. 2008;26(25):4124–30.

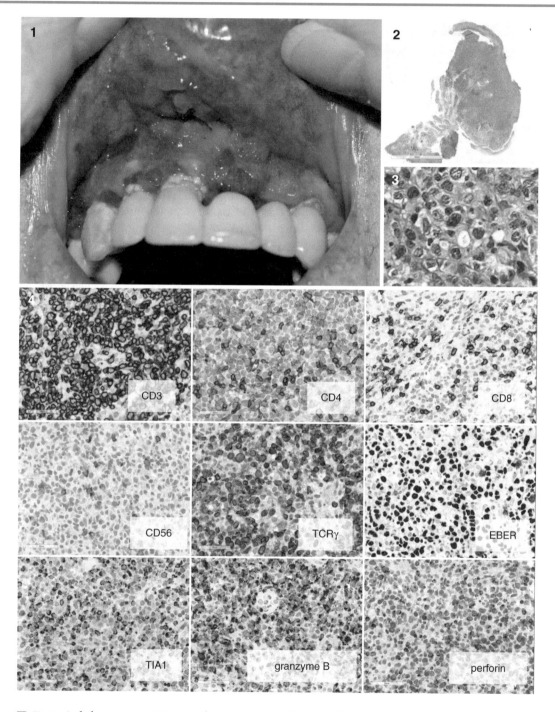

Case 26. Extranodal NK/T-Cell lymphoma, extra-nasal type

F. Dimitriou, M. -C. Brüggen, and E. Guenova

Age: 51   **Sex:** F

Clinical features: The patient presented with a treatment-resistant nodule on her right foreleg. She was otherwise asymptomatic and related the nodule to a mosquito bite a few weeks earlier. Clinical examination showed a solitary erythematous subcutaneous nodule on the right calf, which was firm and painful on palpation. There was no additional cutaneous involvement and no lymphadenopathy. Skin biopsy revealed a small-to-medium sized pleomorphic, highly proliferative CD3+ CD2+ T-cell population with CD8 expression in approximately 30% of all T cells. Skin flow cytometry demonstrated a clearly defined CD16+ CD56+ NK-cell population. Molecular analysis did not detect any clonal rearrangement of the TCR; immunohistochemistry was negative for TCR γ/δ or β-F1 (TCR α/β). EBV in situ hybridization was highly positive. PET-CT excluded nasal involvement and systemic dissemination.

Diagnosis: Extranodal NT/T-cell lymphoma, extra-nasal type.

Follow-up: Following initially successful radiation therapy (6 × 20 Gy), a local relapse occurred. Combined methotrexate + interferon + percutaneous radiotherapy and methotrexate/asparaginase/dexamethasone were ineffective. Following two cycles of SMILE chemotherapy (dexamethasone, methotrexate, ifosfamide, Peg-asparaginase, and etoposide) and an allogeneic HSCT with reduced intensity conditioning, the patient achieved a partial remission of disease. She eventually developed an acute and, subsequently, chronic cutaneous GVHD (superficial sclerosis, lichenoid oral involvement). After 18 months, she died due to disease progression with a massive pericardial effusion with tumor cells.

Comment: ENKTL nasal type manifests mostly in the nasal/paranasal area and can further involve the skin, gastrointestinal tract and, in rare cases, the bone marrow. An extra-nasal manifestation of ENKTL is less common, resulting in the suggestion of some authors that, in most cases of extra-nasal ENKTL, an occult nasal involvement was missed on initial evaluation/staging. Treatment modalities for ENKTL include radiotherapy, chemotherapy, or a combination of both. Allogeneic HSCT is reserved for patients with relapsed/refractory disease. This patient achieved and maintained remission for approximately 18 months.

References

Bruggen MC, Kerl K, Haralambieva E, Schanz U, Chang YT, Ignatova D, et al. Aggressive rare T-cell lymphomas with manifestation in the skin: a monocentric cross-sectional case study. Acta Derm Venereol. 2018;98(9):835–41.

Shet T, Suryawanshi P, Epari S, Sengar M, Rangarajan V, Menon H, et al. Extranodal natural killer/T cell lymphomas with extranasal disease in non-endemic regions are disseminated or have nasal primary: a study of 84 cases from India. Leuk Lymphoma. 2014;55(12):2748–53.

Suzuki R. Pathogenesis and treatment of extranodal natural killer/T-cell lymphoma. Semin Hematol. 2014;51(1):42–51.

Tse E, Kwong YL. The diagnosis and management of NK/T-cell lymphomas. J Hematol Oncol. 2017;10(1):85.

Tse E, Chan TS, Koh LP, Chng WJ, Kim WS, Tang T, et al. Allogeneic haematopoietic SCT for natural killer/T-cell lymphoma: a multicentre analysis from the Asia Lymphoma Study Group. Bone Marrow Transplant. 2014;49(7):902–6.

Fig. 1 Large erythematous firm and painful nodules on the lower extremities. Published with kind permission of © Acta Derm Venereol 2018. All Rights Reserved

Fig. 2 Flow cytometry of the skin biopsy clearly demonstrated a population of CD3− CD16+ CD56 positive cells. Published with kind permission of © Acta Derm Venereol 2018. All Rights Reserved

Fig. 3 Small-to-medium sized pleomorphic, highly proliferative CD3+ CD2+ T-cell population with dim CD8. Published with kind permission of © Acta Derm Venereol 2018. All Rights Reserved

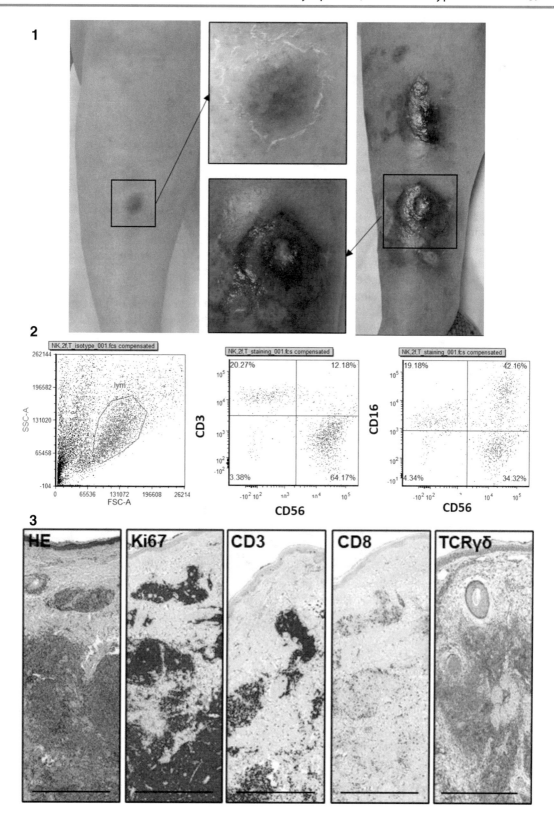

Case 27. Disseminated extranodal NK/T-cell lymphoma

J. Cury-Martins and J. A. Sanches

Age: 47   **Sex:** F

Clinical features: Asymptomatic infiltrated papules, ulcerated nodules and tumors on the abdomen and left lower limb, with rapid growth, for the last 4 months. Presence of a left inguinal adenopathy (1.5 cm). No B symptoms, no complains on the superior aerodigestive tract, no mucosal involvement. Skin biopsy indicated a dense diffuse atypical lympho-histiocytic infiltrate through the entire dermis, with areas of necrosis. Immunohistochemistry and flow cytometry of skin biopsy demonstrated cells positive for CD3, CD56, TIA1, EBV, with high KI67 and negative for CD5, CD30, and TCR rearrangement (by PCR). Laboratory revealed a decrease in the peripheral white blood cell count (3100 µL with 460 lymphocytes), and serum lactate dehydrogenase of 241 IU/L (normal 135–214 IU/L). Bone marrow biopsy showed no involvement. Even though patient had no upper respiratory complains or lesions, PET-CT revealed high intake areas on the skin, inguinal lymph nodes, and nasal mucosa (maxSUV 21.5).

Diagnosis: Disseminated extranodal NK/T-cell lymphoma.

Follow-up: Patient was refractory after two cycles of asparaginase-based chemotherapy (SMILE), with rapid disease progression and death 4 months after diagnosis.

Comment: NK/T-cell lymphomas are extranodal EBV-related malignancies, mostly of NK-cell. Cells are typically positive for CD3 (cytoplasmic), CD56, cytotoxic markers, and EBV. Cases are divided into three subtypes: *Nasal*—the most common (80%), involves the nose, nasopharynx, and the upper aerodigestive tract; *Extra-nasal*—around 20% of cases, involves the skin, gastrointestinal tract, testis, and other sites; *Disseminated*—occurs rarely and involves multiple organs. When cases present in non-nasal sites, PET-CT might help identifying possible occult nasal involvement; if so, patient should be considered as having a disseminated subtype. Regarding treatment, asparaginase-based regimens are currently the standard, with/without radiotherapy. Allogeneic HSCT may be useful in patients with advanced stage and relapsed disease.

References

Tse E, Kwong YL. Diagnosis and management of extranodal NK/T cell lymphoma nasal type. Expert Rev Hematol. 2016;9(9):861–71.

Tse E, Kwong YL. The diagnosis and management of NK/T-cell lymphomas. J Hematol Oncol. 2017;10(1):85.

Tse E, Kwong YL. NK/T-cell lymphomas. Best Pract Res Clin Haematol. 2019;32(3):253–61.

Yamaguchi M, Suzuki R, Oguchi M. Advances in the treatment of extranodal NK/T-cell lymphoma, nasal type. Blood. 2018;131(23):2528–40.

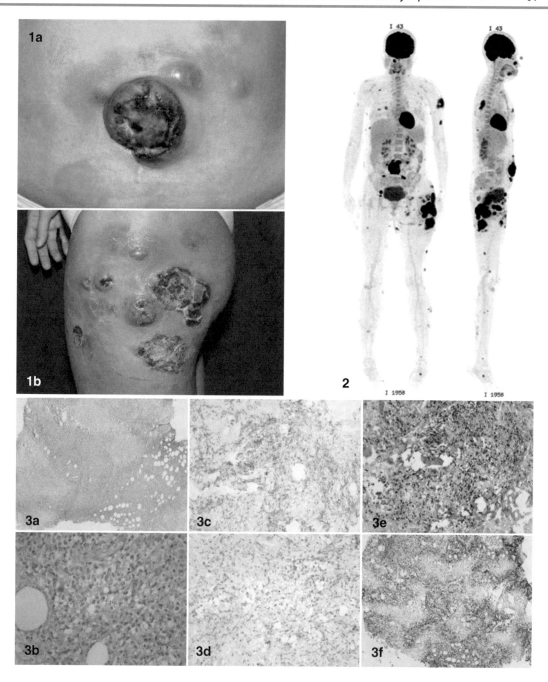

Fig. 1 Nodules, plaques, and tumors (a) on the abdomen and (b) left thigh

Fig. 2 PET-CT revealing (˙) nasal involvement

Fig. 3 Dense atypical lympho-histiocytic infiltrate through dermis and subcutis with necrosis. HE (a) 40×; (b) 400×; (c) CD56, 200×; (d) TIA1, 200×; (e) EBV, in situ hybridization, 200×; (f) Ki67, 40×

γ/δ-Positive T-Cell Lymphomas

Primary cutaneous γδ T cell lymphoma (PCGD-TCL) is characterized by expression of cytotoxic markers and shares clinical features with extranodal NK/T cell lymphoma and primary cutaneous CD8+ aggressive epidermotropic T cell lymphoma. Γδ-positive cases with panniculitis-like presentation should be called as PCGD-TCL with panniculitis-like presentation and not as subcutaneous panniculitis-like T-cell lymphoma with γδ expression. Those cases were shown to originate almost exceptionally from TCR-Vδ2 γδ T cells comprising the separate category. PCGD-TCL has a predilection for extremities and frequently ulcerates. The absence of cytotoxic markers characterizes cases of MF with γδ expression. The cases with EBV+ CD56+ TCRγ+ presents a matter of active debate is that an extranodal NK/T-cell lymphoma with aberrant TCRγ expression or is that a case of EBV+ CD56+ primary cutaneous γδ T cell lymphoma.

Characteristic clinical and immunophenotypic features of various types of primary cutaneous lymphomas expressing TCRγ

Lymphoma	Clinical features	T-cell phenotype	Cytotoxic proteins	Proliferation index (Ki-67)	Major lineage
TCRγ + MF	Classic patches and plaques on extremities	CD3+ CD4+ CD8− CD45RO+ CCR4+	–	Low (10–15)	Memory αβ T cell
PCGD-TCL with MF-like presentation	Ulcerating plaques and tumors	CD3+, CD4−, CD8−/+, CD56+/−, CCR4-	+	High (>50)	γδ T cell
PCGD-TCL with panniculitis-like presentation	Subcutaneous nodules	CD3+, CD4−, CD8+, CD56+	+	High (>50)	γδ T cell
γδ LyP type D	Waxing and waning papulonodules	CD3+ CD30+ CD8+	+	Medium (20–50)	Activated αβ T cell
T-LBL with γδ	Large violaceous nodules in head and neck areas	CD3+, CD5+, CD4+, CD8−, CD56, TdT+	–	High (>50)	Precursor T cell

LyP lymphomatoid papulosis, *PCGD-TCL* primary cutaneous γδ T-cell lymphoma, *T-LBL* T-cell lymphoblastic lymphoma

Case 28. Primary cutaneous γδ T-cell lymphoma with mycosis fungoides-like plaques

B. Rooke, Y. L. Hock, S. Chaganti, and J. Scarisbrick

Age: 44   **Sex:** F

Clinical features: The patient presented with a 33-month history of indurated plaques distributed over the lower limbs and abdomen. No B symptoms were reported. Histology revealed an extensive neoplastic lymphocytic infiltrate involving the epidermis, dermis, and subcutis; epidermotropism and rimming of the fat cells were also seen. Atypical lymphocytes were CD2+, CD3+, CD5−, CD7±, CD56+, CD4−, CD8−, βF1−, and expressed cytotoxic granules TIA1 and perforin. Flow cytometry excluded peripheral blood involvement. PET scan demonstrated cutaneous uptake but no nodal or visceral disease.

Diagnosis: Primary cutaneous γδ T-cell lymphoma.

Follow-up: After two cycles of gemcitabine, her skin disease had progressed. She switched to oral etoposide and achieved partial response after six cycles. Cyclophosphamide, doxorubicin, vincristine, prednisolone, and etoposide (CHOEP-21) are planned. Allogenic hematopoietic stem-cell transplantation will be considered if a complete response is achieved.

Comment: Primary cutaneous γδ T-cell lymphoma arises from a clonal proliferation of cytotoxic T-cells that express cell-surface receptors containing γδ heterodimers. It is very rare, accounting for <1% of all primary cutaneous lymphomas. While immunoreactivity for the TCR-γ subunit can be identified in other cutaneous T-cell lymphomas including MF and lymphomatoid papulosis type D, primary cutaneous γδ T-cell lymphoma can be distinguished by its characteristic CD56+ and βF1− phenotype. The neoplastic lymphocytes may express cytotoxic proteins, show clonal TCR δ gene rearrangement, and are usually CD4−/CD8−, although CD8+ cases are reported. The infiltration pattern correlates with the cutaneous presentation; lesions with epidermotropism present with MF-like patches and thin plaques, and deep dermal or subcutaneous infiltrates present with subcutaneous panniculitis-like indurated plaques or nodules. Lymphoma prefers the limbs with relative sparing of the trunk. It typically has an aggressive course with a 5-year disease-specific survival of 11%. Management is yet to be standardized due to its rarity. Single-agent or multi-agent chemotherapy is often given first line, and it can be combined with superficial radiotherapy. If remission is achieved, allogeneic hematopoietic stem-cell transplantation should be considered in eligible patients to aim for a possible cure.

References

Rodríguez-Pinilla SM, Ortiz-Romero PL, Monsalvez V, et al. TCR-γ expression in primary cutaneous T-cell lymphomas. Am J Surg Pathol. 2013;37:375–84.

Toro JR, Liewehr DJ, Pabby N, et al. Gamma-delta T-cell phenotype is associated with significantly decreased survival in cutaneous T-cell lymphoma. Blood. 2003;101:3407–12.

Vose J, Armitage J, Weisenburger D, et al. International T-Cell Lymphoma Project. International peripheral T-cell and natural killer/T-cell lymphoma study: pathology findings and clinical outcomes. J Clin Oncol. 2008;26:4124–30.

Willemze R, Cerroni L, Kempf W, et al. The 2018 update of the WHO-EORTC classification for primary cutaneous lymphomas. Blood. 2019;133:170–1714.

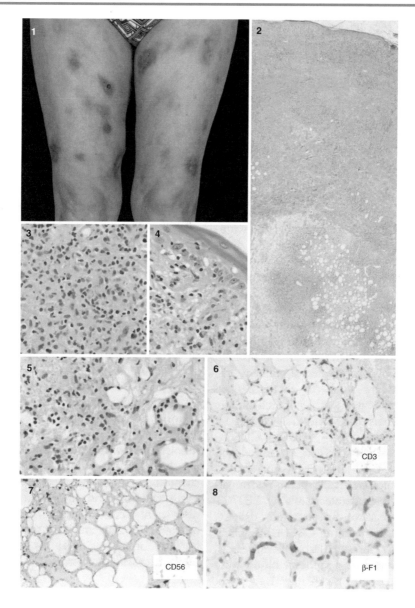

Case 29. Indolent primary cutaneous γδ T-cell lymphoma mimicking mycosis fungoides

X. Martinez, J. Zain, and C. Querfeld

Age: 75 **Sex:** F

Clinical features: The patient presented with numerous scaly, lichenified, erythematous plaques on bilateral arms and upper back. Noted to have a 30-year history of chronic dermatitis, which was initially sparse and asymptomatic, but became pruritic and widespread over time. The patient was also diagnosed with ulcerative colitis at age 18, which was complicated by colon cancer, requiring total colectomy and adjuvant chemotherapy and radiation. Her skin process was initially diagnosed as psoriasis and treated with topical steroids with the initial response but relapsed quickly, and new lesions continued to develop. Biopsies revealed significant epidermotropism by small to medium-sized atypical lymphocytes with hyperchromatic nuclei with irregular contours. Neoplastic cells were CD3+, CD4−, CD8−, CD56−, weakly positive for perforin, had reduced expression of CD2 and CD7, and had a TCRγδ+ phenotype. TCR gene rearrangement studies demonstrated clonality. PET/CT scans were negative for systemic disease. Laboratory tests including CBC, CMP, LDH, flow cytometry for circulating Sézary cells, and TCR analysis in peripheral blood were within normal limits or were negative.

Diagnosis: Primary cutaneous γδ T-cell lymphoma (PCGD-TCL).

Follow-up: A combination of skin-directed and systemic therapy was initiated with the use of daily topical steroids, topical mechlorethamine 0.016% gel three times a week, and subcutaneous injections of interferon-α 1 mln IU three times a week. At a 2-month follow-up, the patient was tolerating treatment and had achieved a partial response.

Comment: PCGD-TCL is a rare disease, comprising <1% of all primary cutaneous lymphomas. It most commonly presents with papules, plaques, and/or nodules with a tendency to ulcerate and having an aggressive clinical course and poor prognosis. Involvement of the oral mucosa, gastrointestinal tract, and/or liver may be seen, but metastasis to lymph nodes and bone marrow is rare. Indolent forms with psoriasis- or MF-like, scaly erythematous patches and plaques have been reported. The development of PCGD-TCL is linked to autoimmunity arising from γδ T cells responsible for regulating immune responses. Neoplastic cells are predominantly small- to medium-sized with elongated or irregular nuclei, are CD2+, CD3+, CD4−, CD8−, CD5−, CD7+/−, and TCR-δ+, and express cytotoxic proteins (TIA1, granzyme B, perforin). Rare CD4+ or CD8+ cases have been documented. EBV is generally negative. Indolent cases may be treated with skin-directed regimens, similar to MF. Multi-agent chemotherapy, followed by allogeneic stem cell transplantation is recommended for aggressive disease. Interferons, retinoids/rexinoids, methotrexate, radiation, and most recently, brentuximab vedotin for CD30+ disease have been used with varied success.

References

Foppoli M, Ferreri AJ. Gamma-delta t-cell lymphomas. Eur J Haematol. 2015;94(3):206–18.

Guitart J, Weisenburger DD, Subtil A, Kim E, Wood G, Duvic M, et al. Cutaneous gammadelta T-cell lymphomas: a spectrum of presentations with overlap with other cytotoxic lymphomas. Am J Surg Pathol. 2012;36(11):1656–65.

Rubio-Gonzalez B, Zain J, Garcia L, Rosen ST, Querfeld C. Cutaneous gamma-delta T-cell lymphoma successfully treated with brentuximab vedotin. JAMA Dermatol. 2016;152(12):1388–90.

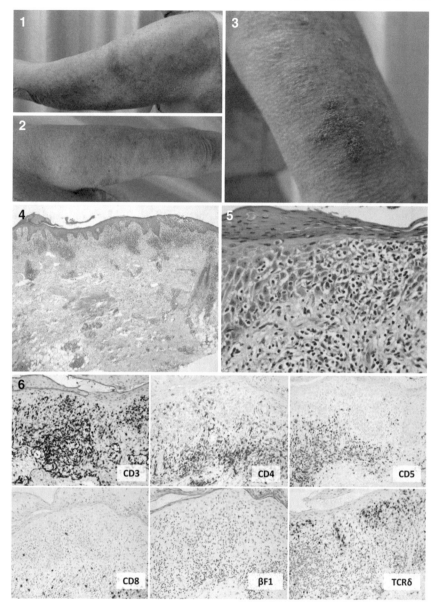

Case 30. Primary cutaneous T-cell lymphoma with gamma/delta (γδ) phenotype: MF or indolent type of gd?

M. Koumourtzis, L. Marinos, and E. Papadavid

Age: 57   **Sex:** M

Clinical features: The patient presented with a 4-year history of multiple violet-to-red patches, and plaques. The original biopsy was consistent with plaque MF. The initial treatments involved PUVA and topical steroids with partial response. He continued to have a progressive skin disease with multiple relapses. The repeated biopsy showed a population of CD8+ γδ T cells, and the patient was diagnosed with primary cutaneous γδ T-cell lymphoma. He was treated with CHOEP (six sessions), autologous stem cell transplantation (BEAM), chemotherapy with gemcitabine (four sessions), local radiotherapy, and very potent topical steroids (near CR). The repeat skin biopsy showed atypical lymphoid infiltrate of small-to-medium size cells, involving the epidermis and dermis, consisting of CD3+CD4−CD5−CD8+CD56− cells with a strong expression of TCRγ+ and a high Ki-67 of 60–70%. The absence of large atypical cells in the biopsy and the absence of systemic involvement made MF's diagnosis with a γδ phenotype most likely. We initiated TSEB with a partial but short-term response. The next treatment was PEG-Interferon alpha-2a, but the disease progressed.

Diagnosis: Indolent primary cutaneous γδ T-cell lymphoma or MF with a γδ phenotype showing an aggressive course.

Follow-up: The patient progressed with multiple violaceous infiltrated plaques. He received treatment with pegylated doxorubicin (45 mg) with an initial partial response. After the sixth cycle, his disease had started to progress again. He is now being planned for allogeneic hematopoietic stem cell transplantation.

Comment: Primary cutaneous γδ T-cell lymphoma (PCγδTCL) is a rare and usually aggressive lymphoma, with a 5-year survival only 11%. However, the earlier reports have identified a few cases associated with a more protracted and even indolent course. The expression of TCRγδ has also been found in rare cases of otherwise classic MF or LyP. These cases can be clinically and histopathologically similar, and the way that these lymphomas should be classified either as a more indolent variant of PCγδTCL or MF with γδ phenotype remains to be clarified. In conclusion, identification of a γδ phenotype in a case clinically and histopathologically resembling MF requires a close follow-up and awareness of potential aggressive behavior.

References

Kempf W, Kazakov DV, Scheidegger PE, Schlaak M, Tantcheva-Poor I. Two cases of primary cutaneous lymphoma with a γ/δ + phenotype and an indolent course: further evidence of heterogeneity of cutaneous γ/δ + T-cell lymphomas. Am J Dermatopathol. 2014;36:570–7.

Khallaayoune M, Grange F, Condamina M, Szablewski V, Guillot B, Dereure O. Primary cutaneous gamma-delta T-cell lymphoma: not an aggressive disease in all cases. Acta Derm Venereol. 2020;100(1):adv00035.

Merill ED, et al. Primary cutaneous T-cell lymphomas showing gamma-delta (γδ) phenotype and predominantly epidermotropic pattern are clinicopathologically distinct from classic primary cutaneous γδ T-cell lymphomas. Am J Surg Pathol. 2017;41:204–15.

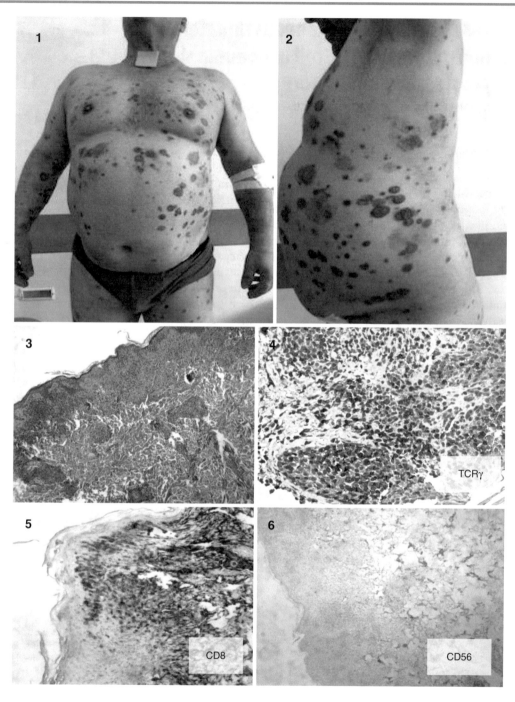

■ **Figs. 1–2** Multiple violet-to-red patches and plaques

■ **Fig. 3** Dermis and epidermis infiltrated by atypical cells. H&E, ×10

■ **Fig. 4** Expression of TCRγ+ cells

■ **Fig. 5** Atypical cells are positive for CD8+

■ **Fig. 6** Negative CD56 expression

Case 31. Primary cutaneous unilateral non-cytotoxic γδ T-cell lymphoma slowly progressing into tumors

L. Huseinzad, J. Ho, and O. E. Akilov

Age: 75 years   **Sex:** M

Clinical features: The patient initially presented with persistent red patches and papules on the right foot only. Initial biopsy revealed a dense band-like lymphocytic infiltrate at the dermo-epidermal junction with epidermotropism, with diminished CD2 and CD5, and prominent γδ T-cells. Molecular studies confirmed a monoclonal population. Peripheral blood flow cytometry was negative. The patient responded to external radiation therapy and oral bexarotene 375 mg, which he discontinued after 1 year due to peripheral edema. Remained clear on topical mechlorethamine until the disease recurrence 2 years after the diagnosis, the disease progressed to an ulcerated tumor on the plantar surface of the right foot, treated with intralesional triamcinolone with rapid resolution of the tumor. He was managed with comprehensive wound care for the healing of the foot ulcers, but a year later again developed a tumor on the right foot and patches and plaques on the right leg. He was treated with local electron beam therapy for his tumor, restarted on NB-UVB, and oral bexarotene 150 mg, with rapid resolution of all lesions within 1 month.

Diagnosis: Primary cutaneous unilateral non-cytotoxic γδ T-cell lymphoma

Follow up: Six months later, the patient developed several sub-centimeter nodules on the right thigh, foreleg, and dorsal surface of the right foot. Repeat biopsy revealed similar findings along with scattered CD30 positivity within the dermis and epidermis, and mild positivity of TIA-1. The therapy with brentuximab vedotin was initiated.

Comment: The differential diagnostics of primary cutaneous γδ T-cell lymphoma from γδ subtype of MF is very challenging and sometimes requires a long-term monitoring the disease pathomorphosis and course. The γδ subtype of MF is rare, with only a few cases in the literature, and characterized by expression of monoclonal γδ T-cell receptor (TCRγδ). Importantly, γδ-MF has been observed to have an indolent course with clinical findings similar to classical MF. Localization of lymphoma exceptionally on the extremity, re-occurrence of tumors, re-gaining the expression of cytotoxic marker (TIA-1) allows us to classify this case as primary cutaneous γδ T-cell lymphoma rather than γδ-MF.

References

Prillinger KE, Trautinger F, Kitzwögerer M, Eder J. Two faces of gamma-delta mycosis fungoides: before and after renal transplantation. BMJ Case Rep. 2017;2017:bcr2016216990.

Rodríguez-Pinilla SM, Ortiz-Romero PL, Monsalvez V, Tomás IE, Almagro M, Sevilla AG, Longo MI, Pulpillo A, Diaz-Pérez JA, Montes-Moreno S, Castro Y, Echevarría B, Trébol I, Gonzalez C, Sánchez L, Otín AP, Requena L, Rodríguez-Peralto JL, Cerroni L, Piris MA. TCR-γ expression in primary cutaneous T-cell lymphomas. Am J Surg Pathol. 2013;37(3):375–84.

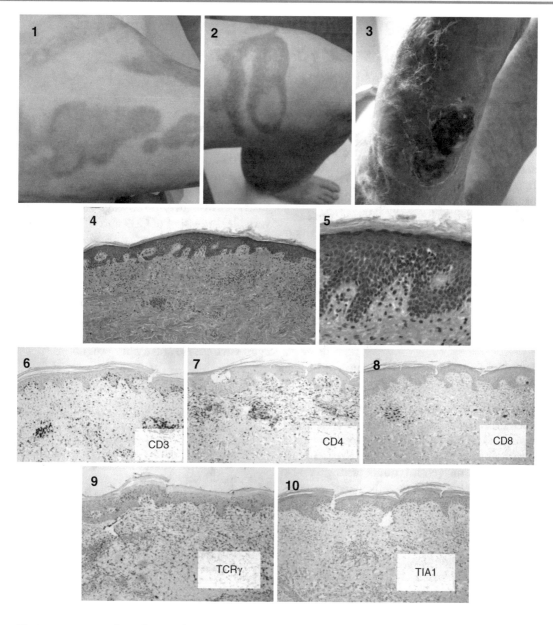

■ **Figs. 1 and 2** Polycyclic coalescing annular red patches with central clearing on the right thigh

■ **Fig. 3** Tumor on the plantar surface of the right sole

■ **Fig. 4** Sparse superficial infiltrate of small-to-medium size lymphocyte. HE, ×20. Published with kind permission of © Jonhan Ho 2019. All Rights Reserved

■ **Fig. 5** The epidermotropism of atypical lymphocytes. HE, ×40. Published with kind permission of © Jonhan Ho 2019. All Rights Reserved

■ **Figs. 6–10** The atypical lymphocytes are CD3+ γδ TCR+, CD4−, CD8−, TIA1−. Published with kind permission of © Jonhan Ho 2019. All Rights Reserved

Case 32. Primary cutaneous γδ T-cell lymphoma with panniculitis-like presentation

M. Koumourtzis, L. Marinos, and E. Papadavid

Age: 60   **Sex:** F

Clinical features: A 60-year-old woman presented with multiple subcutaneous nodules non-responsive to topical steroids. Physical examination revealed multiple subcutaneous nodules located on her right anterior trunk and tights. All nodules were surgically excised, and a complete workup including the whole-body CT scan, bone marrow biopsy, and PET/CT scan was performed, revealing no extracutaneous involvement of lymphoma. Skin biopsy showed γδ T-cell lymphoma positive for CD2, CD3, and TCRγ, and negative for CD4 and CD8 involving the subcutaneous fat only.

Diagnosis: Subcutaneous panniculitis-like T-cell lymphoma with γδ phenotype.

Follow-up: The patient received treatment with chemotherapy (CHOP) and was examined regularly in our specialized center for cutaneous lymphomas and rare diseases. She had an excellent and uneventful course, lasting 6 years, until she developed new subcutaneous nodules, showing the disease recurrence.

Comment: PCGDTCL is a rare and usually aggressive lymphoma, with a 5-year survival only 11%, but some cases run an indolent course. Patients usually present with sometimes ulcerated or necrotic plaques, nodules, and tumors, located on limbs and trunk. Histopathological analysis usually displays an atypical lymphoid infiltrate, involving the epidermis, dermis, or subcutis. Immunohistochemical analysis typically displays CD3+CD4−CD5− TCRαβ− TCRγ+CD8− medium to large-size cells with variable expression of CD7 and CD56. A trend toward a favorable outcome was noted for patients with subcutaneous fat involvement compared with other patients who also had the epidermal and dermal disease. Such PCGDTCL cases with a chronic indolent course are rare, and only a few have been reported, challenging the fact that PCGDTCL always shows an aggressive course and a poor prognosis.

References

Kempf W, Kazakov DV, Scheidegger PE, Schlaak M, Tantcheva-Poor I. Two cases of primary cutaneous lymphoma with a γ/δ + phenotype and an indolent course: further evidence of heterogeneity of cutaneous γ/δ + T-cell lymphomas. Am J Dermatopathol. 2014;36:570–7.

Khallaayoune M, Grange F, Condamina M, Szablewski V, Guillot B, Dereure O. Primary cutaneous gamma-delta T-cell lymphoma: not an aggressive disease in all cases. Acta Derm Venereol. 2020;100(1):adv00035.

Merill ED, et al. Primary cutaneous T-cell lymphomas showing gamma-delta (γδ) phenotype and predominantly epidermotropic pattern are clinicopathologically distinct from classic primary cutaneous γδ T-cell lymphomas. Am J Surg Pathol. 2017;41:204–15.

Fig. 1 Subcutaneous nodules on the patient's tights

Fig. 2 The epidermis and dermis are not infiltrated by atypical cells. H&E, ×10

Fig. 3 Dense infiltration in the subcutaneous fat. HE, ×10

Fig. 4 Expression of TCRγ+ cells. TCRαβ−

Fig. 5 The atypical cells are CD3 positive

Fig. 6 The atypical cells are CD4 negative

Fig. 7 The atypical cells are CD8 negative

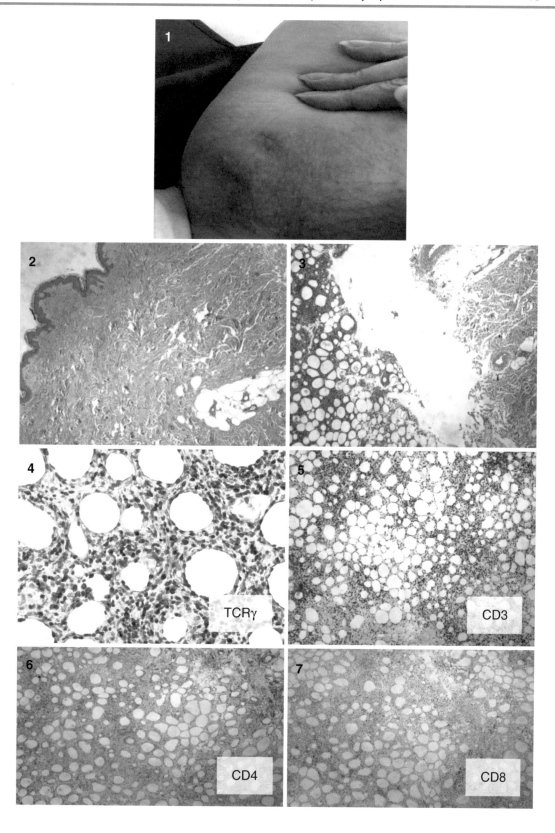

VI

CD8+ Cytotoxic

CD8 marker is not unique to primary cutaneous aggressive epidermotropic CD8+ cytotoxic T-cell lymphoma (pc CD8[+] AECTCL). Moreover, it occurs in seven other entities presented in the following table. There is a certain clinical and morphological overlap of γδ-positive and CD8-positive cases. Due to various aberrant expression of CD56, TCRγ, and CD8 markers, it was suggested that the term "primary cutaneous aggressive epidermotropic cytotoxic T-cell lymphoma" without specification may be better suited for those lymphomas. There is a range of CD8+ pseudolymphomas and CD8+ non-lymphomatous proliferations should be kept on a list of differential diagnosis such as actinic reticuloid, CD8+ drug-associated eruptions, and HIV-associated CD8+ LPD.

Characteristic clinical and immunophenotypic features of various types of primary cutaneous lymphomas expressing CD8 (modified from Willemze R, Cerroni L, Kempf W, et al. The 2018 update of the WHO-EORTC classification for primary cutaneous lymphomas. *Blood.* 2019;133(16):1703–1714)

Lymphoma	Clinical features	T-cell phenotype	Cytotoxic proteins	Major lineage
pc CD8[+] AECTCL	Ulcerating plaques, nodules, and tumors	CD3+, CD4−, CD8+ CD45RA+	+	Naïve αβ T cell
SPTCL	Subcutaneous nodules	CD3+, CD4−, CD8+	+	αβ T cell
Acral CD8[+] T-cell lymphoma	Solitary papule or nodule on acral site (ear, nose)	CD3+, CD4−, CD8+, CD68+	+/−[a]	αβ T cell
CD8+ MF	Hypopigmented patches in kids and young adults	CD3+ CD4+ CD8+ CD45RO+ CCR4+	−	Memory αβ T cell
CD8+ LyP type D	Waxing and waning papulonodules	CD3+ CD30+ CD8+	+	Activated αβ T cell
PCGD-TCL	Ulcerating plaques and tumors	CD3+, CD4−, CD8−/+, CD56+ CCR4-	+	γδ T cell
Extranodal NK/T-cell lymphoma	Ulcerating plaques and tumors	CD3+, CD4−, CD8+ (surface CD3−), CD56+, EBV+	+	NK/T cell
CD8+ T-PLL	Elderly with B symptoms and facial erythema	CD3+, CD4+/− CD5+, CD7+, CD8+, CD52+	−	αβ intermediate T cell

LyP lymphomatoid papulosis; *PCGD-TCL* primary cutaneous γ/δ T-cell lymphoma, *SPTCL* subcutaneous panniculitis-like T-cell lymphoma, *CD8+ T-PLL* CD8+ T-cell prolymphocytic leukemia
[a]Expresses a nonactivated cytotoxic phenotype, positive for TIA-1, but negative for other cytotoxic proteins

Case 33. Primary cutaneous aggressive epidermotropic CD8-positive T-cell lymphoma with initial protracted course

M. H. Trager, C. Magro, and L. J. Geskin

Age: 82   **Sex:** F

Clinical features: The patient presented with a 5-month history of pruritic red patches that started on the back. After a period of stable disease, the patches rapidly progressed to plaques and tumors. The biopsy revealed extensive infiltration of the epidermis and adnexal structures by atypical lymphocytes with a striking degree of syringotropism. The infiltrate exhibited vasocentricity with supervening injurious vascular alterations. Atypical lymphocytes had a distinctive non-cerebriform appearance and were predominately small and intermediate sized with a minor large cell component (<30%) without evidence of CD30 positivity. The atypical cells were CD8-positive and expressed cytotoxic markers (granzyme B and TIA); there was preservation of CD7 and loss of CD2 expression. The CD4 stain was negative. Flow cytometry was negative for blood involvement. PET/CT showed multifocal FDG-avid cutaneous and bilateral lower extremity intramuscular lesions and cervical, axillary, and pelvic lymphadenopathy.

Diagnosis: Primary cutaneous aggressive epidermotropic CD8-positive T-cell lymphoma (pcAETCL) with CD30-large cell transformation (Berti's Lymphoma).

Follow-up: Pralatrexate and bexarotene were initiated. Pralatrexate was discontinued after six cycles due to disease progression. She was subsequently enrolled onto the anti-CD47 clinical trial (Trillium Therapeutics, TTI-621) but passed away shortly thereafter.

Comment: Patients with pcAETCL have a sudden onset of patches, plaques, and nodules. This is in contrast to the gradual evolutionary course seen with MF. In an initial series by Berti et al., patients with pcAETCL had frequent involvement of the oral mucosa and metastatic spread to the testis, lungs, and central nervous system, but lymph node involvement was uncommon. None achieved complete remission with any therapies including PUVA, IFN-α, retinoids, total skin electron beam irradiation, chemotherapy, or allogenic bone marrow transplant. All patients with pcAETCL died within 14–50 months after diagnosis. The spectrum of primary cutaneous CD8+ aggressive epidermotropic T-cell lymphomas has since been expanded to include a protracted variant (similar to MF). In one series, a subset of patients had a prodromal phase of chronic patch stage disease before developing the aggressive ulcerative lesions. It is possible that our patient would fit into this category of patients with the protracted prodromal phase as she had developed patches 5 months prior to rapid disease progression.

References

Berti E, Tomasini D, Vermeer MH, et al. Primary cutaneous CD8-positive epidermotropic cytotoxic T cell lymphomas. A distinct clinicopathological entity with an aggressive clinical behavior. Am J Pathol. 1999;155:483–92.

Guitart J, Martinez-Escala ME, Subtil A, et al. Primary cutaneous aggressive epidermotropic cytotoxic T-cell lymphomas: reappraisal of a provisional entity in the 2016 WHO classification of cutaneous lymphomas. Mod Pathol. 2017;30:761–72.

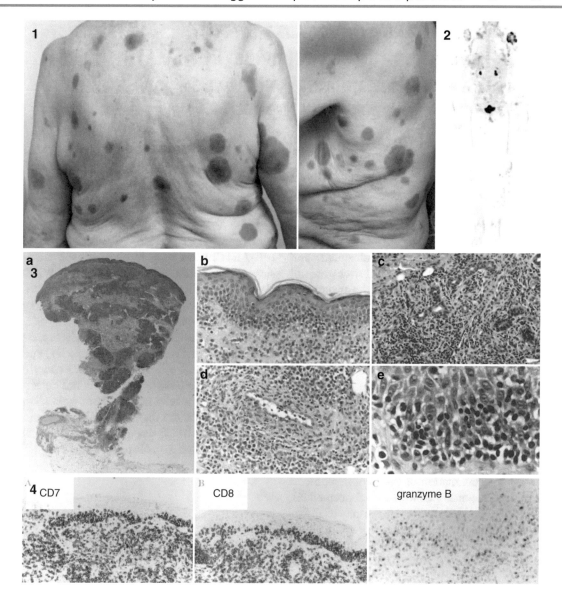

■ Fig. 1 Patches and plaques on initial presentation

■ Fig. 2 PET/CT scan

■ Fig. 3 A striking epidermotropic and pandermal lymphocytic infiltrate. The infiltrate assumes a multinodular growth pattern in the dermis exhibiting accentuation around adnexal structures and blood vessels (**a**). The extensive colonization of the basilar and parabasilar portions of the epidermis (**b**). The extensive infiltration of the adnexal structures by malignant lymphocytes (**c**). There is prominent infiltration of blood vessels by atypical lymphocytes (**d**). The atypical cytomorphology is appreciated; however, the cells are distinctly non-cerebriform in nature (**e**)

■ Fig. 4 The extensive highlighting of the infiltrate for CD7 (**a**). The lymphocytes are of the CD8 subset (**b**). The lymphocytes express granzyme (**c**)

Case 34. Primary cutaneous aggressive epidermotropic T-cell lymphoma (PC-AETCL) with an aberrant immune phenotype

F. DIMITRIOU, M. -C. BRÜGGEN, AND E. GUENOVA

Age: 69 **Sex:** Female

Clinical features: The patient presented with a 3-month history of weight loss and night sweats. Clinically, multiple, sharply demarcated targetoid erythematous patches and plaques were found on the trunk and extremities, most of them centrally ulcerated, and painful upon palpation. Mucosal sites were not involved. A skin biopsy revealed a prominent lymphocytic infiltrate exhibiting an aberrant cytotoxic phenotype. The tumor cells were negative for CD4, CD30, CD7 and CD56, and EBV (EBER1) with low CD8, but high expression of the cytotoxic molecules perforin and granzyme B. TCR genotyping revealed two clonal fragments (201/202 and 204/205 bp). Chromosomal translocation analysis was unremarkable.

Diagnosis: PC-AETCL with an aberrant immune phenotype.

Follow-up: Examination of the peripheral blood and the bone marrow showed no abnormalities, and a total body computer tomography (CT) further excluded extracutaneous organ involvement. Skin-directed treatment with class IV topical corticosteroids and disinfectant bathes remained ineffective. Administration of bexarotene (300 mg/day) and methotrexate (20 mg/week) combined with local radiotherapy resulted in partial healing of the lesions. Two months later, she developed generalized, painful, centrally necrotic plaques. Following one cycle of pegylated liposomal doxorubicin (20 mg/m²),

her condition deteriorated. She developed an extensive oral candidiasis, fever, leukocytopenia, and hyperchromic macrocytic anemia. She died from sepsis 93 days after the initial diagnosis.

Comment: Primary cutaneous CD8+ aggressive epidermotropic cytotoxic T-cell lymphoma (PC-AETCL) has been recognized as a provisional entity in the 2016 revision of the WHO classification of lymphoid neoplasms. The prototypic immunophenotype of this lymphoma entity is CD3+/CD4−/CD8+ with monoclonal rearrangement of the TCR gene. Tumor cells express cytotoxic molecules (TIA-1+, granzyme B+) and the α/β-TCR. NK cell markers (CD56) and γ/δ TCR are not expressed, and EBV is not detectable, in neoplastic cells. In some cases, expression of pan-T-cell-markers may be lost. As also seen in this case, PC-AETCL has an aggressive clinical course with an unfavorable prognosis.

References

Berti E, Tomasini D, Vermeer MH, Meijer CJ, Alessi E, Willemze R. Primary cutaneous CD8-positive epidermotropic cytotoxic T cell lymphomas. A distinct clinicopathological entity with an aggressive clinical behavior. Am J Pathol. 1999;155(2):483–92.

Bruggen MC, Kerl K, Haralambieva E, Schanz U, Chang YT, Ignatova D, et al. Aggressive rare T-cell lymphomas with manifestation in the skin: a monocentric cross-sectional case study. Acta Derm Venereol. 2018;98(9):835–41.

Swerdlow SH, Campo E, Pileri SA, Harris NL, Stein H, Siebert R, et al. The 2016 revision of the World Health Organization classification of lymphoid neoplasms. Blood. 2016;127(20):2375–90.

- **Fig. 1** Sharply demarcated targetoid erythematous patches and plaques were found on the trunk. Published with kind permission of © Acta Derm Venereol 2018. All Rights Reserved
- **Fig. 2** Ulcerated nodule. HE, ×2. Published with kind permission of © Acta Derm Venereol 2018. All Rights Reserved
- **Fig. 3** Atypical lymphocytes at the dermo-epidermal junction. HE, ×60. Published with kind permission of © Acta Derm Venereol 2018. All Rights Reserved
- **Fig. 4** Atypical lymphocytes are positive for CD3, perforin, and granzyme B. Published with kind permission of © Acta Derm Venereol 2018. All Rights Reserved

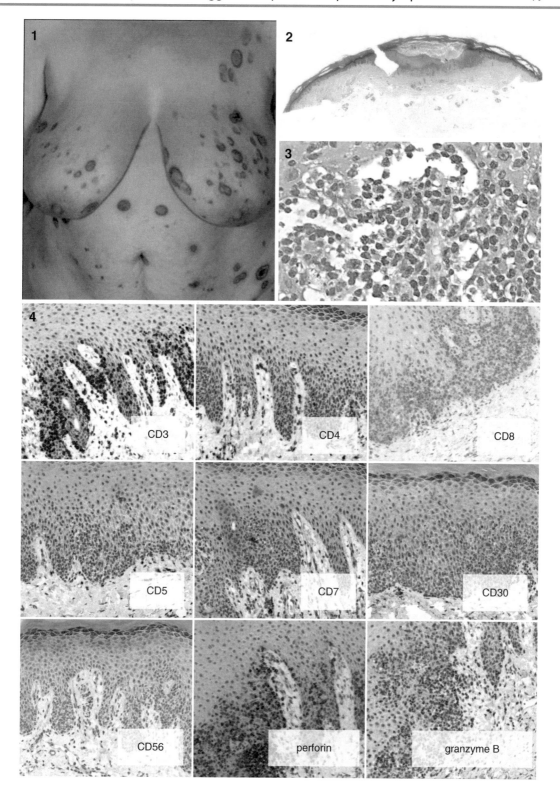

Case 35. CD8+ T-cell lymphoma with cytotoxic phenotype

T. Feldman

Age: 59   **Sex:** M

Clinical features: A homeless alcohol-dependent man developed red nodules over the left flank, which quickly necrotized merging into a large deep ulcer. The patient lost 20 lb and was very fatigued. He developed bacteremia on two occasions. Several skin biopsies showed a dense atypical lymphoid infiltrate spraying into the deep dermis and subcutaneous adipose tissue. The atypical lymphocytes were small-to-medium size with irregular nuclear contours, condensed chromatin, and mostly indistinct nucleoli. Lymphocytes appear to rim adipocytes focally. Immunohistochemical stains show that those atypical lymphocytes were mostly CD3+ CD2+ T-cells that show mild and moderate downregulation of CD5 and CD7, respectively. The majority of these T-cells also co-express CD8, TIA-1, and granzyme B (minor subset) with no evidence of β-F1 expression. Perforin and CD56 were negative. In situ hybridization for EBV mRNA (EBER-ISH) was negative. TCR gene rearrangement study showed a distinct clonal population of T-cells. Comprehensive molecular profile aimed to identify molecular abnormalities in DNA of 177 genes and RNA in 68 genes revealed high expression of CD8 T-cell markers and high expression of PD-L1 mRNA. Laboratory findings: anemia, normal LDH, undetectable EBV DNA in peripheral blood, negative TCR rearrangement, and flow cytometry in peripheral blood, HIV, HTLV1/2 negative. Blood culture, QuantiFERON, ferritin, and sIL2 receptor were normal. Wound and tissue cultures negative. PET scan shows FGD-avid left flank infiltrative lesions.

Diagnosis: Primary cutaneous CD8+ T-cell lymphoma

Follow-up: Patient had minimal response to decadron and started on romidepsin. After two doses, his pain has improved, and no further lesions have developed.

Comments: While primary cutaneous γδ T-cell lymphoma (pcGDTCL) was considered in this patient, the lack of CD56 and TCR-γ expression argues against this diagnosis. Ultimately, a diagnosis of CD8+ cutaneous T-cell lymphoma with cytotoxic expression was rendered as the morphology, and immunophenotype did not fit into a specific WHO-recognized category.

This case reflects the difficulties of establishing the diagnosis. pcGDTCL is an aggressive cutaneous lymphoma of mature, activated γδ T-lymphocytes, accounting for less than 1% of all lymphomas. It tends to present with disseminated plaques and nodules and may develop ulcerations. Mucosal involvement is frequent. However, involvement of lymph nodes, spleen, or bone marrow is uncommon. Morphologically, there are three patterns of cutaneous involvement: epidermotropic, dermal, and subcutaneous. More than one pattern may co-exist in a single biopsy specimen or present in different biopsy specimens from the same patient. pcGDTCL used to be included within subcutaneous panniculitis-like T-cell lymphoma with a γδ phenotype but is now a separately recognized entity due to its more aggressive clinical course. The clinical course is frequently associated with hemophagocytosis and hemophagocytic lymphohistiocytosis (HLH). Median survival is less than 15 months. Optimal therapy is not established, but allogeneic stem cell transplantation appears to be curative in select patients.

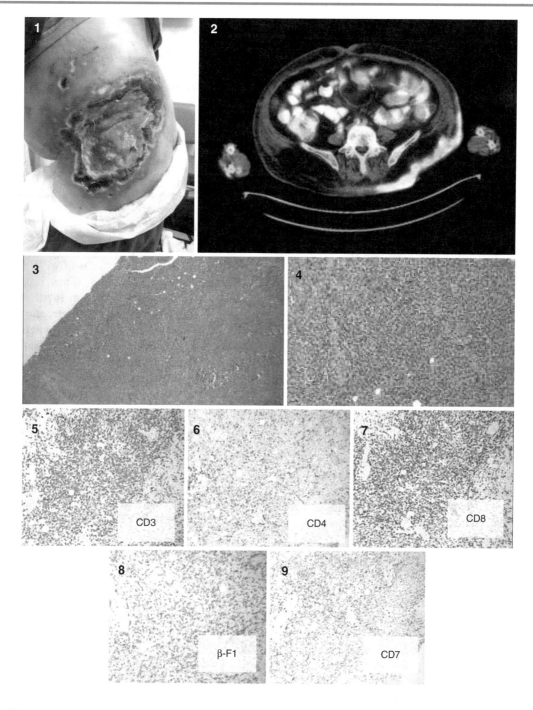

Fig. 1 Large ulcerated mass on the left flank. Published with kind permission of

Fig. 2 PET/CT scan

Fig. 3 Dens lymphocytic infiltrate, HE, ×10

Fig. 4 Sheets of atypical lymphocytes. HE, ×20

Fig. 5 Atypical cells were CD3 positive

Fig. 6 Atypical cells were CD4 negative

Fig. 7 Atypical cells were CD8 positive

Fig. 8 Atypical cells were β-F1 negative

Fig. 9 Atypical cells were CD7 dim

Case 36. Primary cutaneous aggressive epidermotropic T-cell lymphoma as a composite lymphoma with B-cell chronic lymphocytic leukemia

F. Dimitriou, M. -C. Brüggen, and E. Guenova

Age: 56   **Sex:** Male

Clinical features: The patient presented with disseminated ulcerating skin nodules, oral necrotic ulcerations, and axillary and cervical lymphadenopathy. In addition, he had a 2-week history of decreased appetite, weight loss, and night sweats. Six years ago, he was diagnosed with chronic lymphocytic leukemia followed up with watchful waiting. Clinical examination revealed disseminated, painful, centrally ulcerating nodular lesions (up to 5 cm in size), one large oral necrotic plaque and generalized lymphadenopathy. A skin biopsy revealed a CD3+/CD8+/CD4−/TCRβ–F1+ proliferative infiltrate of small atypical lymphocytes accumulating in the perivascular and periadnexal areas. Molecular analysis demonstrated a clonal rearrangement of the TCR. PET-CT scan revealed multiple metabolically active cutaneous and subcutaneous lesions and generalized lymphadenopathy. Histology confirmed further T-cell lymphoma involvement in the lymph nodes and in the bone marrow.

Diagnosis: PC-AETCL as a composite lymphoma with B-cell CLL.

Follow-up: A systemic treatment with R-CHOEP (rituximab, cyclophosphamide, doxorubicin, vincristine, etoposide, and dexamethasone) was initiated. After 6 cycles, he achieved a complete remission, which allowed for a reduced conditioning regimen (fludarabine 30 mg/m², busulfan 4 × 1 mg/kg and ATG 10 mg/kg), and an allogeneic HSCT of a human leukocyte antigen (HLA)-identical donor. The first 9 months of follow-up were uneventful. Afterwards, his CLL relapsed and he then developed a spontaneous bacterial peritonitis with a septic shock and subsequently death.

Comment: PC-AETCL constitute a rare, poorly characterized subgroup of cutaneous lymphoma and are, according to the 2016 WHO classification, still considered as a provisional entity. A recent analysis of data from 34 patients with PC-AETCL confirms poor prognosis, with a 5-year survival rate of 32% and a median survival of 12 months. Autologous/allogeneic HSCT has shown promising results in several recently published cases. This patient achieved a remission of at least 9 months after R-CHOEP and allogeneic HSCT.

References

Bruggen MC, Kerl K, Haralambieva E, Schanz U, Chang YT, Ignatova D, et al. Aggressive rare T-cell lymphomas with manifestation in the skin: a monocentric cross-sectional case study. Acta Derm Venereol. 2018;98(9):835–41.

Guitart J, Martinez-Escala ME, Subtil A, Duvic M, Pulitzer MP, Olsen EA, et al. Primary cutaneous aggressive epidermotropic cytotoxic T-cell lymphomas: reappraisal of a provisional entity in the 2016 WHO classification of cutaneous lymphomas. Mod Pathol. 2017;30(5):761–72.

Plachouri KM, Weishaupt C, Metze D, Evers G, Berdel WE, Kempf W, et al. Complete durable remission of a fulminant primary cutaneous aggressive epidermotropic CD8(+) cytotoxic T-cell lymphoma after autologous and allogeneic hematopoietic stem cell transplantation. JAAD Case Rep. 2017;3(3):196–9.

Swerdlow SH, Campo E, Pileri SA, Harris NL, Stein H, Siebert R, et al. The 2016 revision of the World Health Organization classification of lymphoid neoplasms. Blood. 2016;127(20):2375–90.

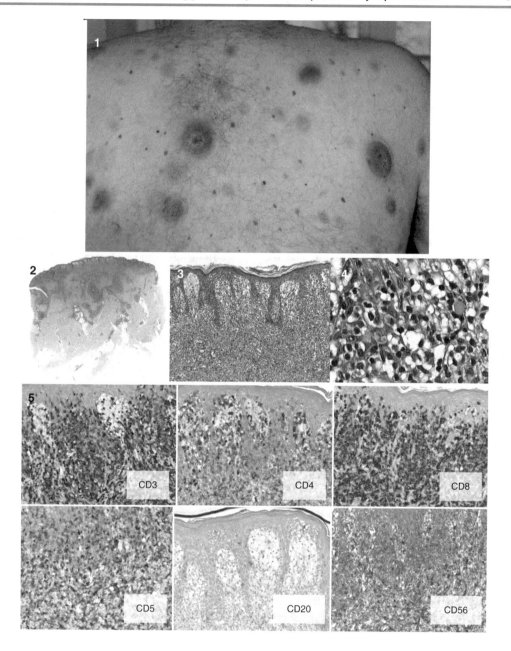

Case 37. Primary cutaneous aggressive epidermotropic CD8+ cytotoxic T-cell lymphoma with bullous manifestation

X. Martinez, J. Zain, and C. Querfeld

Age: 86 **Sex:** F

Clinical features: The patient presented with erythematous nodules on the right earlobe, ill-defined erythematous patches on the face, and painful, erosive, annular, violaceous plaques on the right lower extremity. Biopsy demonstrated an ulcerated epidermis with prominent pagetoid epidermotropism of atypical lymphocytes and a dermal and subcutaneous lymphoid infiltrate composed of atypical, monomorphic lymphocytes. Immunophenotyping revealed a CD3+, CD8+, βF1+, and cytotoxic (weakly CD56+, TIA-1+, granzyme B+, perforin+) phenotype with a high proliferation (Ki67) index of ~70%, negative for CD2, CD4, CD5, CD7, and CD30. TCR showed clonal rearrangement. EBER-ISH was negative. No systemic symptoms or peripheral lymphadenopathy were present. A clonal TCR rearrangement was not detected in the blood. PET/CT scans were negative for systemic disease. The four cycles of pegylated doxorubicin (30 mg/m²) led to complete remission. Relapse occurred with few erythematous, thin plaques, and tense bullae on the right lower extremity. Repeated skin biopsy of the bullous lesion revealed the recurrent disease.

Diagnosis: Primary cutaneous aggressive epidermotropic CD8+ cytotoxic T-cell lymphoma (CD8+ AECTCL)

Follow-up: A cutaneous relapse was managed with high-potency topical steroids and close monitoring for nearly 1 year until additional lesions developed. Pegylated doxorubicin was re-started, but discontinued after three cycles due to lack of response. Palliative radiation was administered for disease control.

Comment: pc CD8+ AECTCL has an unfavorable prognosis with a 5-year overall survival rate of 18–32%. It may clinically present with chronic papules, patches, plaques, or tumors prior to developing an aggressive course with ulcerated/necrotic lesions. Nodal metastases are infrequent with a tendency for systemic spread, specifically lungs, central nervous system, and testes. Characteristic histologic features are a prominent pagetoid, intraepidermal infiltration of monomorphous, atypical lymphocytes and dyskeratotic/necrotic keratinocytes with or without ulceration. Neoplastic T-cells are typically positive for CD3, CD8, CD7, and beta F1, express cytotoxic proteins (TIA-1, granzyme B, perforin), regain features of a naïve T-cell phenotype (CD2−, CD45RA+), and are negative for CD4, CD5, CD45RO, CD30, CD56, and EBER-ISH. Cases with CD4/CD8 double negative phenotype have been described. Patients are typically treated with single- or multi-agent doxorubicin-based chemotherapy. Allogeneic stem-cell transplantation is considered for younger patients and/or those refractory to treatment.

Reference

Guitart J, Martinez-Escala ME, Subtil A, Duvic M, Pulitzer MP, Olsen EA, et al. Primary cutaneous aggressive epidermotropic cytotoxic T-cell lymphomas: reappraisal of a provisional entity in the 2016 WHO classification of cutaneous lymphomas. Mod Pathol. 2017;30(5):761–72.

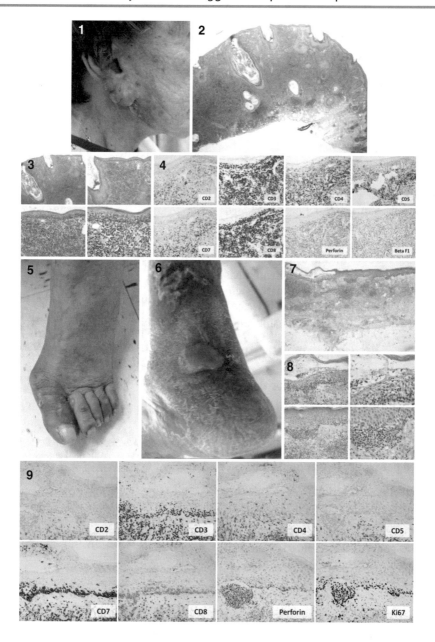

■ Fig. 1 A tumor lesion on earlobe and ill-defined erythematous patch on cheek

■ Fig. 2 A dense, deep, dermal lymphoid infiltrate

■ Figs. 3 and 4 Extensive, full-thickness, pagetoid epidermotropism of medium-sized lymphocytes, and a dense dermal infiltrate of medium-sized, monomorphic, atypical lymphocytes, HE, ×20 and ×40. The tumor cells are positive for CD3, CD8, and βF1, with expression of perforin, and negative for CD2, CD4, CD5, and CD7

■ Figs. 5–8 Clinical presentation of same patient showing erosive plaques and bullae a few months later

■ Fig. 9 An intraepidermal blister with pagetoid epidermotropism of atypical lymphocytes and a superficial, atypical lymphoid dermal infiltrate. Strong CD3, CD8, and perforin expression with preserved CD5 and CD7 expression, negative for CD2 and CD4. The proliferation (Ki67) index is high among epidermotropic T-cells

Case 38. Leukemoid reaction mimicking aggressive epidermotropic CD8+ T-cell lymphoma

M. Matsumoto, A. Huen, J. Ho, and O. E. Akilov

Age: 49   **Sex:** M

Clinical features: A patient hospitalized for acute pancreatitis secondary to alcohol use complicated by multiorgan dysfunction developed fever, marked leukocytosis (WBC 52.2×10^9/L), and erythroderma with acral purpura 4 weeks into admission. Blood, sputum, urine, and stool cultures were negative. CT of abdomen/pelvis demonstrated diffuse lymphadenopathy and pancreatitis. The patient was empirically treated with broad spectrum anti-bacterial and anti-fungal coverage. Labs otherwise notable for AST and ALT within normal limits, elevated LDH to 2025. Atypical lymphocytes were seen on peripheral blood smear. Skin biopsies demonstrated a band-like infiltrate of epidermotropic lymphocytes which stained positive for CD8, TIA-1, granzyme B, and βF1. TCR gene-rearrangement PCR (BIOMED-2) from skin biopsy demonstrated polyclonal T-cell population.

Diagnosis: Leukemoid reaction (LR) mimicking CD8+ aggressive epidermotropic T-cell lymphoma (CD8+ AECTCL)

Follow-up: The patient's white blood cell count continued to increase from 52.2 to 93.1 to 131.6. His clinical state deteriorated and he passed 4 days after onset of erythroderma and purpura.

Comment: H&E demonstrated epidermotropic and cytotoxic CD8+ T-cells indistinguishable from CD8+ AECTCL. However, those cells were not clonal based on TCR-GR PCR. CD8+ AECTCL is a rapidly progressive lymphoma with poor prognosis which usually presents with widespread, ulcerated or necrotic plaques and nodules. It usually metastasizes to the CNS, lung, and testes; lymph node and peripheral blood involvement is rare. LR is a marked leukocytosis not caused by hematologic malignancy also with poor prognosis. Range of reported leukocytosis on presentation in one study of LR was $11–139 \times 10^9$/L. Infection, hypersensitivity, and paraneoplastic syndrome are common etiologies. Cutaneous manifestations are variable and related to underlying process such as cutaneous metastases in paraneoplastic LR, morbilliform dermatitis in drug hypersensitivity, and retiform purpura in sepsis.

References

Chakraborty S, Keenportz B, Woodward S, Anderson J, Colan D. Paraneoplastic leukemoid reaction in solid tumors. Am J Clin Oncol. 2015;38(3):326–30.

Introcaso CE, Kim EJ, Gardner J, Junkins-Hopkins JM, Vittorio CC, Rook AH. CD8+ epidermotropic cytotoxic T-cell lymphoma with peripheral blood and central nervous system involvement. Arch Dermatol. 2008;144:1027–9.

Nofal A, Abdel-Mawla MY, Assaf M, Salah E. Primary cutaneous aggressive epidermotropic CD8+ T-cell lymphoma: proposed diagnostic criteria and therapeutic evaluation. J Am Acad Dermatol. 2012;67(4):748–59.

Potasman I, Grupper M. Leukemoid reaction: spectrum and prognosis of 173 adult patients. Clin Infect Dis. 2013;57(11):e177–81.

Sakai C, Takagi T, Oguro M, Tanabe N, Wakatsuki S. Erythroderma and marked atypical lymphocytosis mimicking cutaneous T-cell lymphoma probably caused by phenobarbital. Intern Med. 1993;32(2):182–4.

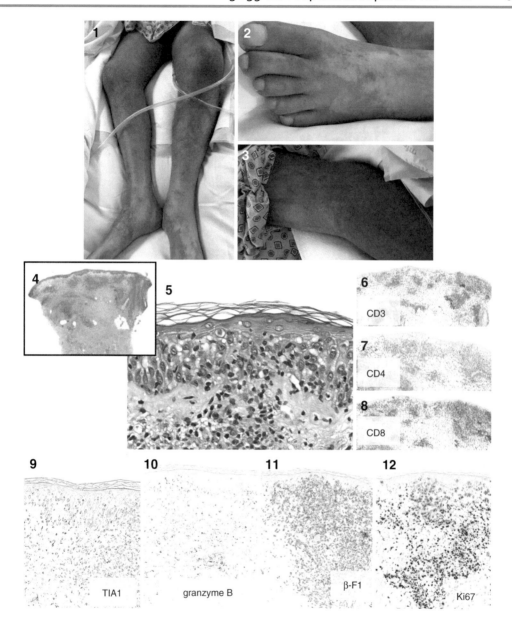

Fig. 1 Bilateral lower extremities with dusky retiform purpura and a few tense fluid filled bullae on the right foot

Fig. 2 Acral purpura

Fig. 3 Retiform purpura around the left knee

Fig. 4 Atypical epidermotropic dense band-like and perivascular infiltrate

Fig. 5 Spongiosis and lymphocytic exocytosis

Fig. 6 Atypical cells positive for CD3

Fig. 7 Atypical cells are negative for CD4

Fig. 8 Atypical cells are positive for CD8

Fig. 9 Atypical cells are positive for TIA1

Fig. 10 Atypical cells are positive for granzyme B

Fig. 11 Atypical cells are positive for βF1

Fig. 12 High Ki67 expression on atypical cells

VII

Peripheral T-Cell

The unusual for MF symmetricity of primary morphological elements is a striking feature of PTCL. PTCL also tends to present with monomorphic granulomatous confluent papulonodules on the upper back, around elbows and knees, which is also quite uncommon for MF. The disproportion of the severity of lymph node involvement (fully effaced) in a patient with "MF IA" disease should render a re-evaluation of "MF as a diagnosis in favor of PTCL." While histological features may significantly overlay with MF, there are several diagnostic features of PTCL, such as high Ki67 (>50%) and an absence of epidermotropism.

Case 39. Cutaneous relapse of peripheral T-cell lymphoma, NOS by extension

C. Vainder, S. Choudhary, J. Ho, and O. E. Akilov

Age: 63 **Sex:** M

Clinical features: The patient with a history of hypertension, diabetes, heart failure with reduced ejection fraction, prolactinoma, and monoclonal gammopathy of undetermined significance was diagnosed with PTCL, NOS a year unrelenting generalized pruritus. The patient was erythrodermic, had generalized lymphadenopathy (completely effaced lymph nodes on histology), and a leukemic blood count. No visceral involvement on PET/CT. The flow cytometry on the peripheral blood and histological evaluation of the right subclavicular lymph node showed that atypical cells of small-to-medium size were positive for CD2, CD3dim, CD4, TCR-$\alpha\beta$, CD5, CD16/CD57, PD-1dim and negative for CD7, CD8, CD26, and CD56. EBER was negative. The patient started on methotrexate and bexarotene, shortly due to low efficacy, ECP was added to control his blood involvement. Two months after, the previous therapies were discontinued, and romidepsin 14 mg/m^2 was started. Due to thrombocytopenia, romidepsin was frequently delayed or administrated in a low dose (7.5–10 mg/m^2). During cycle 3 of romidepsin (10 mg/m^2) due to progression in the blood, alemtuzumab 5 mg SQ was initiated. The patient received LEBT to inguinal lymph nodes and started prednisone taper 60–40–20 mg PO daily over 3 months, achieving CR in the skin for 4 months. However, during cycle 7 of romidepsin, the patient has started developing new monomorphic violaceous patches in bilateral axillae and groin above the involved lymph nodes.

Diagnosis: Cutaneous relapse of peripheral T-cell lymphoma, NOS by extension.

Follow-up: The romidepsin was restarted at 18 mg/m^2. Due to the disease progression, romidepsin was discontinued 2 months later. The patient was started on pralatrexate 15 mg/m^2 on days 1, 8, and 15 in combination with bexarotene 300 mg/m^2 and mechlorethamine gel. A month later, bexarotene was discontinued. A month later, romidepsin 10.5 mg/m^2 was added to pralatrexate 15 mg/m^2 to administer together every 14 days. Radiation to axillary and inguinal lymph nodes was restarted. The patient achieved complete clearance of his skin and overall disease control lasting for 7 months. Two weeks after the last infusion of pralatrexate and romidepsin, the patient was hospitalized with profound weakness, generalized malaise with decreased appetite and nausea. The patient had also noted an increase in balance issues/falls over the last few months: falling multiple times per week. No acute infarct, new hemorrhage or mass effect was on MRI. In the setting of splenic sequestration and multifactorial renal failure, the decision was made to proceed with hospice care, all drugs were discontinued, and the patient died the next day.

Comment: Peripheral T-cell lymphoma is characterized by symmetric monomorphic patches and plaque that are frequently present in axillae and groin. Moreover, the cutaneous relapse of PTCL frequently occurs in the skin about the lymph nodes. The treatment is difficult. Some success was reported with a combination of pralatrexate with romidepsin, which we found helpful for our patient. Unfortunately, significant comorbidity complicated the course of his PTCL and eventually led to a fatal outcome.

Reference

Amengual JE, Lichtenstein R, Lue J, et al. A phase 1 study of romidepsin and pralatrexate reveals marked activity in relapsed and refractory T-cell lymphoma. Blood. 2018;131(4):397–407.

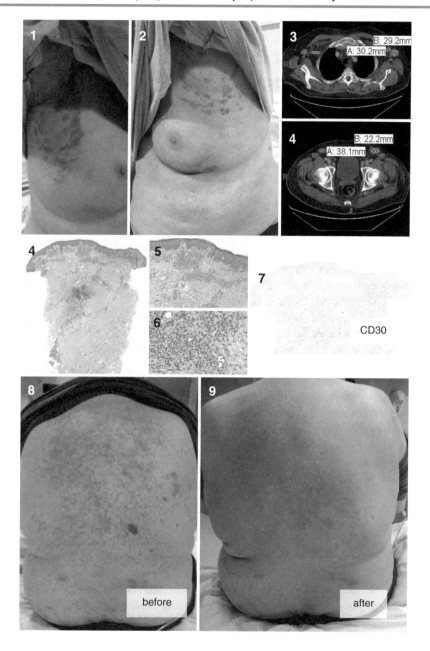

Figs. 1 and 2 Bilateral symmetric violaceous patches in axillae

Figs. 3 and 4 CT shows axillary (Fig. 3) and inguinal (Fig. 4) lymphadenopathy

Figs. 4, 5, and 6 Mildly dense superficial perivascular inflammatory infiltrate composed predominantly of small-to-medium size lymphocytes and histiocytes. Published with kind permission of © Sonal Choudhary 2019. All Rights Reserved

Fig. 7 CD30 negative stain. Published with kind permission of © Sonal Choudhary 2019. All Rights Reserved

Fig. 5 Monomorphic erythematous papulonodules in the mid back prior pralatrexate and romidepsin combination

Fig. 6 Complete clearance after pralatrexate and romidepsin combination

Case 40. Generalized lymphadenopathy and poikiloderma due to prolonged interferon-β-1b Therapy misdiagnosed as peripheral T-cell lymphoma

S. Raychaudhuri, N. Aggarwal, and O. E. Akilov

Age: 83   **Sex:** F

Clinical features: The patient with a history of secondary-progressive multiple sclerosis (MS) was on long-term interferon-β1b therapy for more than 10 years. During the hospital admission for an altered mental status, secondary to upper respiratory infection, CT scan incidentally showed widespread lymphadenopathy involving mediastinal lymph nodes with the largest measuring approximately 3.3 cm. There was no hepatosplenomegaly. The patient did not report any chills, night sweats, or weight loss. A biopsy of the left inguinal lymph node showed complete effacement by polymorphous infiltrate of small lymphocytes, polytypic plasma cells, histiocytes, and occasional large cells. Flow cytometry demonstrated a very high CD4 to CD8 ratio but without a lack of pan T-cell antigens. EBER was negative. The T-cell receptor gene rearrangement demonstrated a clonal pattern. A month later, the patient developed multiple poikilodermatous telangiectatic patches on the chest, back, upper arms, upper back, and face. Biopsy showed the epidermis overlaying a moderately dense, superficial and mid dermal, perivascular, somewhat nodular lymphoid infiltrate composed predominantly of small lymphocytes, histiocytes, and plasma cells. The infiltrate was separated from the epidermis by a Grenz zone. Immunohistochemical studies demonstrated mixed populations of CD3+ T-cells and CD20+ B-cells. A CD4 to CD8 ratio was within the normal range. The expression of CD5 corresponded to the distribution of T-cells. CD30 marked rare scattered cells. Ki-67 proliferation index did not exceed 10% within the infiltrate. T-cell receptor gene rearrangement demonstrated identical clonality to what was detected in the lymph node previously. The IFN-β-1b was discontinued. The poikiloderma resolved within 2 months after discontinuation of IFN-β-1b. A follow-up CT scan of the chest, abdomen, and pelvis was done 9 months later, which showed no residual intrathoracic or intraabdominal lymphadenopathy.

Diagnosis: Pseudolymphoma secondary to prolonged interferon-β1b.

Follow-up: As the lymphadenopathy had resolved completely 9 months after discontinuation of IFN-β-1b, the skin rash and generalized lymphadenopathy were attributed to a lymphomatoid drug reaction and reactive lymphadenopathy due to prolonged IFN-β therapy rather than nodal PTCL with cutaneous involvement despite suggestive pathology and positive T-cell clone in the skin and lymph node.

Comment: Generalized lymphadenopathy mimicking metastatic disease in patients with melanoma treated with IFN-α-2b adjuvant therapy has been published previously. However, poikiloderma and diffuse lymphadenopathy mimicking PTCL, because of long-term IFN-β-1b use for the treatment of MS have never been reported.

References

Cone LA, Brochert A, Schulz K, et al. PET positive generalized lymphadenopathy and splenomegaly following interferon-alfa-2b adjuvant therapy for melanoma. Clin Nucl Med. 2002;32:793–6.

Ridolfi L, Cangini D, Galassi R, et al. Reversible, PET-positive, generalized lymphadenopathy and splenomegaly during high-dose Interferon-α-2b adjuvant therapy for melanoma. J Immunother. 2008;31:675–8.

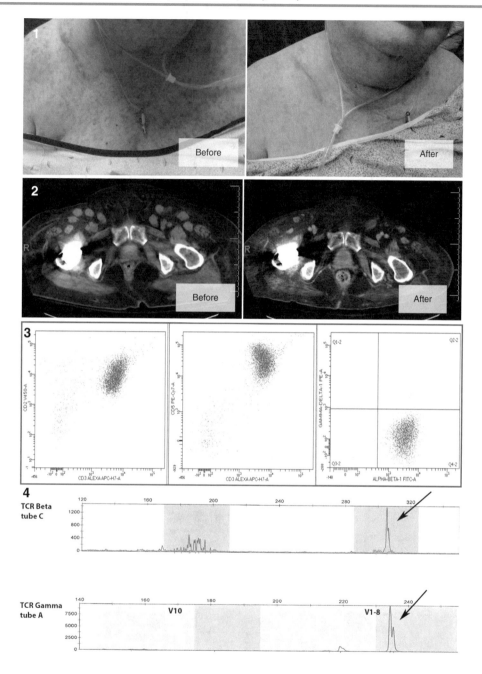

Fig. 1 Multiple poikilodermatous telangiectatic patches on the neck and chest before and after IFN-α-2b

Fig. 2 CT scan showing widespread generalized lymphadenopathy at the initial presentation and resolution of generalized lymphadenopathy after discontinuation of INF-β-1b

Fig. 3 Flow cytometry of the lymph node demonstrated the large population of αβ CD4+ T-cells with preserved CD3, CD5, and CD7 expression. Published with kind permission of © Nidhi Aggarwal 2019. All Rights Reserved

Fig. 4 TCR PCR showed clonal peak. Published with kind permission of © Nidhi Aggarwal 2019. All Rights Reserved

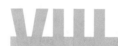

VIII Posttransplant Lympho

Case 41. Cutaneous Epstein–Barr Virus post-transplant lymphoproliferative disorder

G. Dobos, A. de Masson, C. Ram-Wolff, M. Battistella, D. Michonneau, R. Peffault de Latour, P. Brice, and M. Bagot

Age: 40 **Sex:** F

Clinical features: The patient had an 8-year history of Sézary syndrome. She failed multiple lines of therapies including interferon-α combined with extracorporeal photopheresis, bexarotene, mogamulizumab (anti-CCR4), liposomal pegylated doxorubicin, anti-KIR3DL2 monoclonal antibody, a combination of brentuximab vedotin and bendamustine, ifosfamide and etoposide, then gemcitabine, vinorelbine and doxorubicin, both leading to a partial response. Romidepsin and retinoids were not tolerated. The patient was eligible for allogeneic stem cell transplantation from a 10/10 matched unrelated donor and received reduced-intensity conditioning with fludarabine and melphalan, without in vivo T-cell depletion. Both the recipient and the donor had a positive Epstein-Barr virus (EBV) serology before transplantation. After transplantation, the patient had ciclosporin and methotrexate prophylactically to prevent graft-versus-host disease (GvHD). Nevertheless, she developed acute stage 2 cutaneous GvHD and was treated with systemic corticosteroids. Two months after the transplant, the patient presented with reddish erythematous nodules and plaques on the scalp and face and severe pruritus. The biopsy showed an interface dermatitis with a dense pleomorphic lymphocytic infiltration of the dermis with some mature plasma cells. The cells expressed CD20+, PAX5+, MUM1+, CD30+, LMP+, and EBER RNA. The proliferation index Ki67 was 90%. There was no clonal rearrangement of the TCR or IgH/Igk gene detected by PCR in the skin. There was no evidence of nodal disease on the CT scan. The EBV viral load in blood was 2.89 copies/ml.

Diagnosis: Cutaneous polymorphic polyclonal EBV-positive post-transplant lymphoproliferative disorder (PTLD).

Follow-up: The patient received 4 cycles of rituximab 375 mg/m^2 at weekly intervals. The majority of the lesions disappeared after the first infusion. Four additional infusions at monthly intervals were continued as a maintenance treatment. The treatment was well tolerated, and the patient had no evidence of relapse, 6 months after transplantation.

Comment: EBV-positive PTLD occurs after solid organ or allogeneic hematopoietic stem cell transplantation and is a result of the proliferation of EBV-infected cells and a lack of anti-EBV T-cell responses. In the case of allogeneic hematopoietic stem cell transplant, most cases occur in the first year after transplant. If a relapse of cutaneous T-cell lymphoma is suspected after bone marrow transplantation, a biopsy should always be taken. EBV-positive PTLD may present as papules and nodules of the skin. Post-transplant EBV viremia should be monitored by quantitative PCR.

References

Fox CP, Burns D, Parker AN, et al. EBV-associated post-transplant lymphoproliferative disorder following in vivo T-cell-depleted allogeneic transplantation: clinical features, viral load correlates and prognostic factors in the rituximab era. Bone Marrow Transplant. 2013;49:280–6.

Kanakry JA, Hegde AM, Durand CM, et al. The clinical significance of EBV DNA in the plasma and peripheral blood mononuclear cells of patients with or without EBV diseases. Blood. 2016;127:2007–17.

Sanz J, Andreu R. Epstein–Barr virus-associated post-transplant lymphoproliferative disorder after allogeneic stem cell transplantation. Curr Opin Oncol. 2014;26:677–83.

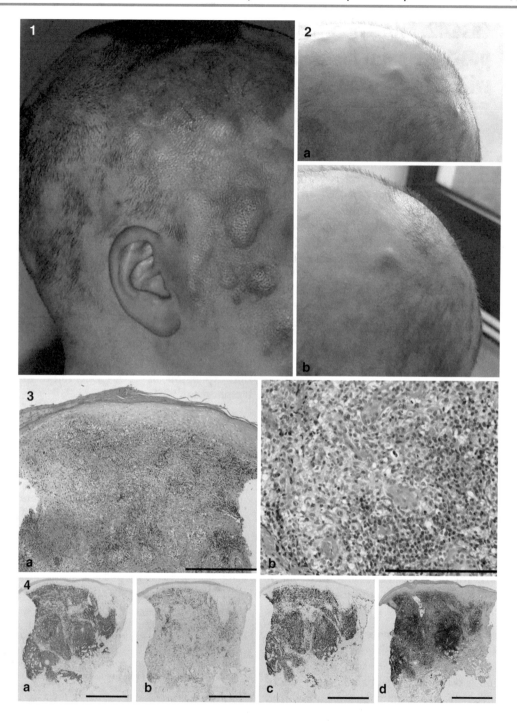

■ Fig. 1 Sézary syndrome with cutaneous large cell transformation prior to bone marrow transplantation

■ Figs. 2 and 3 Erythematous nodules on the scalp of EBV-positive post-transplant lymphoproliferative disorder

■ Fig. 4 Dense dermal infiltrate, HE, ×10

■ Fig. 5 Pleomorphic lymphocytes. HE, ×40

■ Fig. 6 The lymphocytes expressed CD20, but not CD3 with an elevated Ki67 and positive EBER

Case 42. Primary cutaneous CD30 T-cell posttransplant lymphoproliferative disorder with δ expression

V. Kazlouskaya, J. Ho, and O. E. Akilov

Age: 77 **Sex:** F

Clinical features: The patient underwent a liver transplant after primary biliary cirrhosis 17 years ago was on tacrolimus. Three years ago, she developed several red papules on the back that was biopsied and diagnosed as CD30 positive lymphoproliferative disorder. Later, several papules appeared on the thighs, back, neck, and upper extremities along with 3 cm nodule on the left shoulder. The biopsy showed diffuse infiltrate composed of atypical lymphocytes. The cells diffusely expressed CD3, CD30, and δ and were mostly negative for CD2, CD4, CD8, CD5, CD7, CD20, ALK-1, CD56, granzyme B, EBER, and TIA-1. Molecular studies were positive for T-cell rearrangement. Imaging did not reveal any distant metastases.

Diagnosis: Primary cutaneous CD30+ T-cell monomorphic monoclonal posttransplant lymphoproliferative disorder (PTLD) with δ expression.

Follow-up: UVB, topical and intralesional steroids were tried with no improvement. One dose of brentuximab vedotin was given which provided the complete resolution of all her lesions. The maintenance therapy was continued with a low dose of methotrexate with disease control over the last 2 years.

Comment: Although cutaneous γδ T-cell lymphoma was initially considered in our case due to the diffuse strong expression of TCRδ, this diagnosis was not favored based on the lack of characteristic histopathological features and benign course over the years. Γδ T-lymphocytes may be seen in small percentages in benign inflammatory conditions, but their numbers usually do not exceed 10–15% of the infiltrate.

γδ expression in large numbers of the infiltrating cells was reported in a few cases of lymphomatoid papulosis and pityriasis lichenoides. In almost all cases, the same cells were also positive for CD8 and were epidermotropic, with only one case with double negative phenotype CD4−/CD8− similar to our case. It was suggested that CD30+ PTLD has a worse prognosis compared to similar lymphomas in the general population and that gamma-delta phenotype, in general, may be associated with significantly decreased survival in T-cell lymphomas of the skin. Thus, in our case, the unusual expression of TCRδ may be the aberrant expression on CD30+ cells rather than a lymphoma of γδ T-cells.

References

Aalaibac M, Morris J, Yu R, Chu AC. T lymphocytes bearing the gamma delta T-cell receptor: a study in normal human skin and pathological skin conditions. Br J Dermatol. 1992;127:458–62.

Martinez-Escala ME, Sidiropoulos M, Deonizio J, Gerami P, Kadin ME, Guitart J. γδ T-cell-rich variants of pityriasis lichenoides and lymphomatoid papulosis: benign cutaneous disorders to be distinguished from aggressive cutaneous γδ T-cell lymphomas. Br J Dermatol. 2015;172:372–9.

Seçkin D, Barete S, Euvrard S, Francès C, Kanitakis J, Geusau A, Del Marmol V, Harwood CA, Proby CM, Ali I, Güleç AT, Durukan E, Lebbé C, Alaibac M, Laffitte E, Cooper S, Bouwes Bavinck JN, Murphy GM, Ferrándiz C, Mørk C, Cetkovská P, Kempf W, Hofbauer GF. Primary cutaneous posttransplant lymphoproliferative disorders in solid organ transplant recipients: a multicenter European case series. Am J Transplant. 2013;13:2146–53.

Toro JR, Liewehr DJ, Pabby N, Sorbara L, Raffeld M, Steinberg SM, Jaffe ES. Gamma-delta T-cell phenotype is associated with significantly decreased survival in cutaneous T-cell lymphoma. Blood. 2003;101:3407–12.

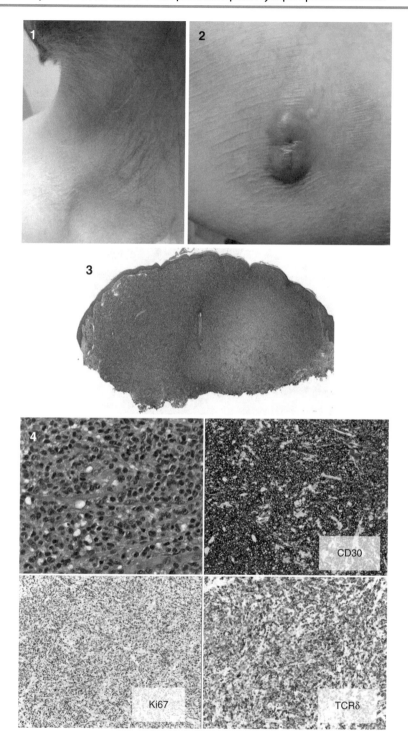

■ Fig. 1 Erythematous papules on the back of the neck

■ Fig. 2 Large nodule on the left shoulder

■ Fig. 3 Diffuse nodular proliferation of neoplastic cells

■ Fig. 4 Higher magnification demonstrating atypical lymphocytic infiltrate composed of small to medium cells diffusely expressing CD30; Ki-67 reflecting high proliferative rate; diffuse positivity cells for TCRδ

IV

Cutaneous B-Cell

Case 43. Primary cutaneous marginal zone lymphoma presented as facial patches unresponsive to rituximab

V. Kazlouskaya, J. Ho, and O. E. Akilov

Age: 55   **Sex:** M

Clinical features: The patient developed asymptomatic violaceous patches and on the temples, cheeks, and upper back. Otherwise, the patient was doing well and had no lymphadenopathy, splenomegaly, or any systemic symptoms. Biopsy of the lesion demonstrated deep nodular folliculotropic infiltrate containing atypical lymphocytes admixed with plasma cells. The infiltrate was predominantly CD20 positive. CD10 and Bcl-6 were not expressed in the germinative centers, while Bcl-2 expression was seen. B-lymphocytes demonstrated predominant λ expression. IgH rearrangement detected clonality of the infiltrate. Bone marrow biopsy and imaging did not demonstrate systemic involvement with lymphoma. Due to the multifocal distribution of the lesions, treatment with rituximab was started. Patient was given 22 courses of rituximab 375 mg/m^2 with no response. Trial of topical imiquimod, thalidomide, valproic acid, and amoxicillin were not successful as well. Localized electron beam therapy 4 Gy in two fractions was subsequently started and resulted in complete resolution of the lesions.

Diagnosis: Primary cutaneous marginal zone lymphoma (PCMZL) presented as facial patches.

Follow-up: The patient remains to be free of patches 3 years after radiotherapy.

Comment: PCMZL is an indolent type of B-cell lymphoma typically presenting as violaceous papules or nodules on the trunk or upper extremities. Associations with viral, bacterial, or autoimmune conditions are known. The treatment of PCMZL is usually conservative. Surgical excision is appropriate for isolated nodules. Other treatment options may include antibiotics, rituximab, radiotherapy, and chemotherapy, but frequently PCMZL recurs. Rituximab was shown to be highly effective for PCMZL in few small studies and case reports, with all cases achieving complete resolution or improvement, and no refractory cases were previously documented. Rituximab resistance mechanisms are multifactorial and may be explained by immunological mechanisms or inefficient metabolism process.

References

Hoefnagel JJ, Vermeer MH, Jansen PM, Heule F, Van Voorst Vader PC, Sanders CJ, Gerritsen MJ, Geerts ML, Meijer CJ, Noordijk EM, Willemze R. Primary cutaneous marginal zone B-cell lymphoma: clinical and therapeutic features in 50 cases. Arch Dermatol. 2005;141:1139–45.

Senff NJ, Noordijk EM, Kim YH, Bagot M, Berti E, Cerroni L, Dummer R, Duvic M, Hoppe RT, Pimpinelli N, Rosen ST, Vermeer MH, Whittaker S, Willemze R. European Organization for Research and Treatment of Cancer and International Society for Cutaneous Lymphoma consensus recommendations for the management of cutaneous B-cell lymphomas. Blood. 2008;112:1600–9.

Valencak J, Weihsengruber F, Rappersberger K, Trautinger F, Chott A, Streubel B, Muellauer L, Der-Petrossian M, Jonak C, Binder M, Raderer M. Rituximab monotherapy for primary cutaneous B-cell lymphoma: response and follow-up in 16 patients. Ann Oncol. 2009;20:326–30.

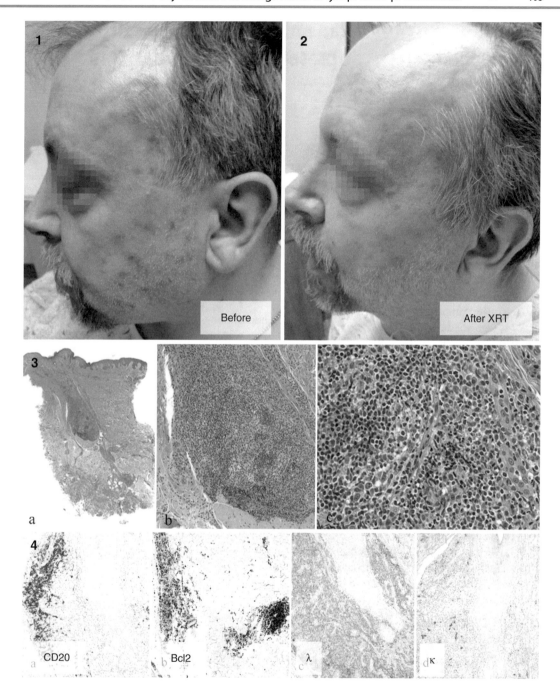

■ Fig. 1 Violaceous patches in the temple areas and cheeks before treatment

■ Fig. 2 Follow-up photograph after treatment with local radiotherapy

■ Fig. 3 Nodular bottom heavy infiltrate with centrocytes and plasma cells. Published with kind permission of © Viktoryia Kazlouskaya 2019. All Rights Reserved

■ Fig. 4 The infiltrate of atypical cells was positive for CD20, Bcl-2 with λ predominant cells over κ expressing cells. Published with kind permission of © Viktoryia Kazlouskaya 2019. All Rights Reserved

Case 44. Primary cutaneous diffuse large B-cell lymphoma, leg type presenting on the scalp

M. O'Donnell, J. Cha, and N. Nikbakht

Age: 72 **Sex:** M

Clinical features: The patient presented with a tender, pink to skin-colored tumor that abruptly appeared on his scalp and in four weeks grew to 4 × 4 cm in size. He denied any constitutional symptoms. Laboratory investigations demonstrated normal peripheral white blood cell count and serum lactate dehydrogenase level and increased beta-2 microglobulin (4.36 mg/L). Although there was an elevated Epstein–Barr virus nuclear antibody (227 U/mL) in the blood, the Epstein–Barr virus genome was not detected in the lesional skin by a polymerase chain reaction. PET scan showed a hypermetabolic left parietal scalp lesion with no other significant uptake. Bone marrow biopsy did not show any evidence of lymphoma. Skin biopsy demonstrated a sheet-like diffuse dense infiltrate composed of centroblasts and immunoblasts with high mitotic activity. The atypical lymphocytes stained positive for CD20, MUM1, BCL6, BCL2, and weakly positive for CD10. Fluorescent in-situ hybridization (FISH) test revealed a positive gene rearrangement for BCL6 (18%) and negative rearrangements for MYC, CCND1, and BCL2. A dominant immunoglobulin heavy chain (IgH) sequence was identified by next generation sequencing with the frequency of 99.999% of all nucleated cells in the skin lesion.

Diagnosis: Primary cutaneous diffuse large B-cell lymphoma, leg type (PCDLBCL, LT).

Follow-up: The patient was a poor candidate for chemotherapy due to comorbidities and underwent local radiation therapy of the scalp lesion (4500 cGy in 25 fractions) with a complete resolution of scalp tumor. The repeat PET scan showed no evidence of the disease.

Comment: It is crucial to differentiate PCDLBCL, LT from other PCBCLs as it is the most aggressive form of PCBCL, carries a different prognosis, and requires a different therapeutic approach. The final diagnosis of PCDLBCL, LT depends on the expressions of CD20, MUM1, BCL2, and in most cases, BCL6 but not CD10 by the large, atypical lymphocytes with a diffuse pattern of distribution. PCFCL and PCMZL stain negative for MUM1, highlighting the importance of MUM1 for proper diagnosis. PCDLBCL, LT commonly disseminates into extracutaneous sites, affects older women, and presents with rapidly growing tumors on the lower legs. Approximately 10–20% of cases may involve other cutaneous sites. Patients with tumors on the lower legs more commonly have extracutaneous involvement than those with lesions elsewhere (33% vs. 18%). Gene rearrangements of MYC, BCL6, and IgH are common with the rearrangements in MYC occurring in 30% of PCDLBCL, LT cases. The MYC gene's rearrangements, especially in combination with the second hit of BCL6 and/or BCL2, are adverse prognostic factors in PCDLBCL, LT.

References

Schrader AMR, Jansen PM, Vermeer MH, Kleiverda JK, Vermaat JSP, Willemze R. High incidence and clinical significance of MYC rearrangements in primary cutaneous diffuse large B-cell lymphoma. Leg Type Am J Surg Pathol. 2018;42(11):1488–94.

Wilcox RA. Cutaneous B-cell lymphomas: 2019 update on diagnosis, risk stratification, and management. Am J Hematol. 2018;93(11):1427–30.

Willemze R, Cerroni L, Kempf W, et al. The 2018 update of the WHO-EORTC classification for primary cutaneous lymphomas. Blood. 2019;133(16):1703–14.

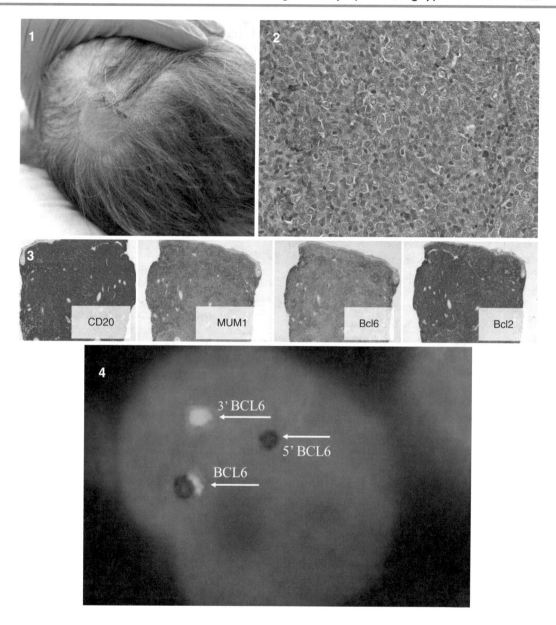

■ Fig. 1 Erythematous nodule on left parietal scalp

■ Fig. 2 Dense infiltration of centroblasts and immunoblasts in the dermis. HE, ×100

■ Fig. 3 CD20, MUM1, BCL6, BCL2 expressions of the infiltrating cells. ×20

■ Fig. 4 FISH test identifying a BCL6 rearrangement

Case 45. Primary Cutaneous Diffuse Large B Cell Lymphoma, Leg Type (PCDLBCL-LT) Treated with Bcl-2 Inhibitor, Venetoclax

F. Abdulla and S. Rosen

Age: 85   **Sex:** Male

Clinical features: Asymptomatic erythematous to violaceous nodules on right lower extremity and few on the left lower extremity appeared abruptly over a month prior to presentation (Fig. 1) without B symptoms. A skin biopsy showed a dense, diffuse, and deep lymphoid infiltrate composed of atypical large lymphocytes with pleomorphic nuclei, finely dispersed chromatin and prominent nucleoli extending into the subcutaneous fat tissue (Fig. 3). Atypical lymphocytes were strongly positive for CD19, CD20, BCL2, MUM1, and cMYC (98%) with a high proliferation index of 95%, partially positive for PD1 representing an activated B cell (ABC) phenotype. BCL2 was also strongly positive (Fig. 4). EBER was negative. FISH showed clonal copy number gains of *MYC* and *BCL2*. *MYD88* was not mutated. Whole-body PET/CT excluded any lymph node or visceral involvement.

Diagnosis: Primary cutaneous diffuse large B cell lymphoma, leg type (PCDLBCL-LT)

Follow up: At diagnosis the localized lesions were treated with radiotherapy, resulting in a partial response. At disease progression, he was treated with R-CGOP with gemcitabine with a partial response that was short in duration. Subsequent disease was treated with pegylated doxorubicin/rituximab, without benefit. The patient was subsequently started on rituximab 375 mg/m² once weekly for the first 4 weeks. Lenalidomide (10 mg/day, days 1–21) was added by the second rituximab administration and 1 month later pembrolizumab was started. This triple combination was repeated every 3 weeks for two cycles. He achieved complete remission and continued receiving lenalido-mide, rituximab and pembrolizumab on a monthly basis for an additional six months. However, the patient subsequently developed new lesions on the right lower extremity. Whole-body PET/CT showed no lymph node or visceral involvement. Because BCL-2 was positive, the patient was initiated on venetoclax. After one cycle, the patient had a complete response of all cutaneous lesions (Fig. 2). However, the patient passed away a month after response due to complications related to his cirrhosis with associated ascites secondary to prior alcohol use and hepatitis B.

Comment: PCDLBCL-LT is an aggressive malignancy with a 5-year overall survival of 50%. The high level of Bcl-2 expression in cases of PCDLBCL-LT suggests that a Bcl-2 inhibitor such as venetoclax may provide a therapy option without major toxicities. In the CAVALLI study, venetoclax in combination with R-CHOP resulted in improved progression-free survival in BCL2-positive subgroups. There is a single reported case in the literature of successful use of venetoclax in PCDLBCL *MYD88* wild-type, chemotherapy- and radiotherapy-refractory PCDLBCL-LT. This is the second reported case.

References

Morschhauser S, Feugier P, Flinn IW, et al. Venetoclax plus rituximab, cyclophosphamide, doxorubicin, vincristine and prednisolone (R-CHOP) improves outcomes in BCL2-positive first-line diffuse large B-cell lymphoma (DLBCL): first safety, efficacy and biomarker analyses from the phase II CAVALLI study. Blood. 2018;132(Suppl 1):782.

Walter HS, Trethewey CS, Ahearne MJ, Jackson R, Jayne S, Wagner SD, Saldanha G, Dyer MJS. Successful treatment of primary cutaneous diffuse large B-cell lymphoma leg type with single-agent venetoclax. JCO Precis Oncol. 2019;3:1–5.

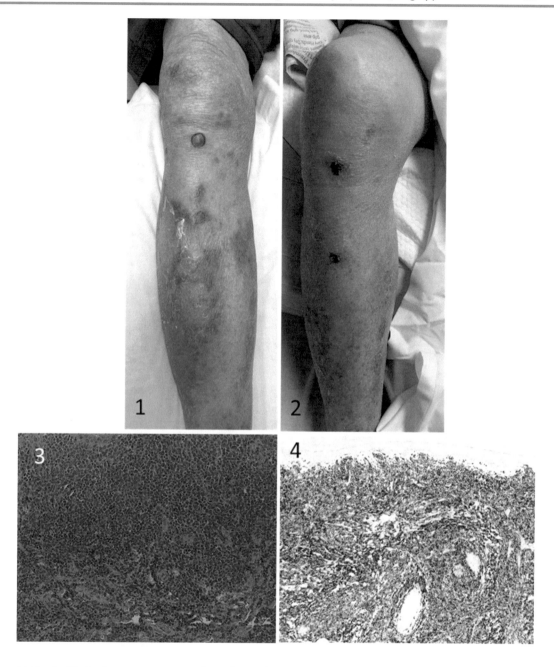

■ Fig. 1 Clinical presentation with indurated red nodules on the right leg and plaques

■ Fig. 2 Clinical regression after the administration of venetoclax

■ Fig. 3 A dense diffuse lymphoid infiltrate composed of atypical large lymphocytes

with large nuclei, finely dispersed chromatin, and prominent nucleoli

■ Fig. 4 Large tumor cells are positive for BCL2

Blastic Plasmacytoid

Blastic plasmacytoid dendritic cell neoplasm (BPDCN) is a rare, aggressive hematologic malignancy primarily in elderly males. Almost all patients present with cutaneous tumors characterized by purpuric hue secondary to thrombocytopenia. Lymphadenopathy and pancytopenia are noted to have varying degrees, and CNS involvement is seen in up to 30% of cases. BPDCN arises from plasmacytoid dendritic cells. Those are large cells typically positive for CD4, CD56, BDCA-2, CD123, and TCL1 and negative for markers of myeloid, T-lymphoid, B-lymphoid, or monocyte lineage. Up to 10–20% of patients with BPDCN have a concurrent history of hematologic malignancy, including myelodysplastic syndrome, chronic myelomonocytic leukemia, and acute myeloid leukemia. BPDCN often undergoes a leukemic transformation with a median survival of less than 1 year. A new subset of skin-limited BPDCN with an excellent prognosis was recently defined; however, it is not clear which patient will remain to have a skin-limited disease since cases of metastatic spread after a presentation with an isolated cutaneous nodule were also described.

Case 46. Bruise-like nodules of blastic plasmacytoid dendritic cell neoplasm on the background of diffuse petechiae

L. Huseinzad, S. Choudhary, J. Ho, and O. E. Akilov

Age: 64   **Sex:** M

Clinical features: The schizophrenic patient presented with asymptomatic red-purple nodules on a background of diffuse petechiae abruptly appeared on the trunk and generalized to the entire body within 1 month, with accompanying weight loss, fatigue, and somnolence. Generalized lymphadenopathy was present on the physical examination. Laboratory investigation was significant for macrocytic anemia, neutropenia, thrombocytopenia, and elevated serum lactate dehydrogenase level (299 U/l, normal 140–271 U/l). Circulating blast cells were positive for CD4, CD26, CD33, CD38, CD123 and HLA-DR, and negative for CD16 and CD30. CD56 expression was weakly present. Bone marrow biopsy showed hypercellular bone marrow with decreased hematopoiesis and extensive involvement (71%) by CD123+ blastic plasmacytoid dendritic cells. Histology revealed a plasmacytic dendritic cell neoplasm positive for CD123, CD56, and CD4, and negative for CD20, CD35, and CD68. The patient declined PET/CT.

Diagnosis: Blastic plasmacytoid dendritic cell neoplasm (BPDCN).

Follow up: Planned for the enrollment into Tagraxofusp-erzs clinical trial. However, the patient refused all treatment and entered hospice care, expiring within 3 months of initial presentation.

Comment: Conventional chemotherapies and stem cell transplantation have been associated with poor efficacy and high rates of relapse/death in patients with BPDCN. Tagraxofusp-erzs (Elzonris, Stemline), a cytotoxin targeting CD123 expressing cells, was approved for the treatment of BPDCN in 2018. Clinical trials revealed an overall response rate of 90%, with the majority being complete remission, and survival rate of 59% at 18 months, which is higher than with conventional chemotherapy. Toxicities include capillary leak syndrome, hepatotoxicity, and hypersensitivity reactions. Tagraxofusp-erzs represents the first FDA-approved treatment for BPDCN, with improved survival compared to existing chemotherapies.

References

Pemmaraju N, Lane AA, Sweet KL, Stein AS, Sumithira V, Blum W, Rizzieri DA, Wang ES, Duvic M, Sloan JM, Spence S, Shemesh S, Brooks CL, Balser J, Bergstein I, Lancet JE, Kantarjian HM, Konopleva M. Tagraxofusp in blastic plasmacytoid dendritic-cell neoplasm. N Engl J Med. 2019;380:1628–37.

Venugopal S, Zhou S, El Jamal SM, Lane AA, Mascarenhas J. Blastic plasmacytoid dendritic cell neoplasm-current insights. Clin Lymphoma Myeloma Leuk. 2019;19(9):545–54.

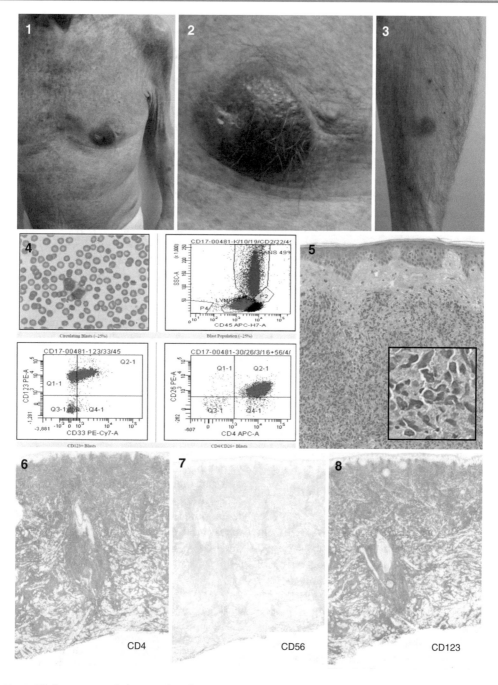

Fig. 1 Violaceous nodules on the chest on a background of diffuse petechiae

Fig. 2 Close-up of the ulcerated tumor on the left chest originally referred to dermatologist as "a cyst"

Fig. 3 Bruise-like nodule on the left foreleg

Fig. 4 Peripheral smear with large plasmacytoid blasts. Flow cytometry of the peripheral blood cells demonstrates presence of CD4+CD123+ blasts

Fig. 5 Dense infiltration of atypical monomorphic medium sized blast cells in the dermis extending into the subcutis. HE. ×20. An insert shows blasts in the dermis with smudged nuclei. HE, ×100

Fig. 6 Blasts are positive for CD4

Fig. 7 Blasts had dim CD56 expression

Fig. 8 Blasts are positive for CD123

Case 47. Blastic plasmacytoid dendritic cell neoplasm presenting with deep purple nodules

A. N. BUI, A. A. LANE, AND N. R. LEBOEUF

Age: 79   Sex: M

Clinical features: The patient presented with a non-healing wound after Moh's surgery for a squamous cell carcinoma in situ on the left frontal scalp. Physical examination showed a crusted, violaceous deep ulceration with punched out borders and surrounding deep purple edematous plaque on the left frontal scalp, an infiltrated plaque with a scar on the right preauricular cheek, and significant swelling on the lateral face extending down onto the anterior trunk. Histopathology showed dense dermal infiltrate of intermediate sized mononuclear cells with irregular to folded nuclei, distinct to prominent nucleoli, and moderate amounts of eosinophilic cytoplasm, positive for CD123, TdT, and negative for CD34. Bone marrow biopsy showed a high grade primitive hematopoietic malignancy with IDH2 c.418G>A p.R140W mutation detected by molecular analysis. Laboratory tests were significant for pancytopenia.

Diagnosis: Blastic plasmacytoid dendritic cell neoplasm (BPDCN).

Follow-up: Treatment was initiated with an IDH2 inhibitor with partial response of BPDCN in the blood but with progression of cutaneous lesions. Palliative radiation therapy (RT) to the cutaneous BPDCN lesions for 20 Gy in five fractions resulted in a partial response in treated areas. The patient was started on combination chemotherapy with doxorubicin, vincristine, and dexamethasone, which was discontinued due to infection. Then, he was treated with Tagraxofusp which provided a partial response of cutaneous lesions at 2 weeks' follow-up. However, his disease progressed. Venetoclax was started next with a weekly dose escalation to 400 mg daily. At 4 weeks, the patient demonstrated a marked response in the skin, a decrease in the size of lymph nodes, but with no bone marrow response. Two weeks later, the patient died from an intracranial hemorrhage.

Comment: Although clinical trials are ongoing, there is a lack of guidelines on the management of BPDCN. There is recently an increase in the use of immunomodulatory agents and novel targeted drugs. Tagraxofusp, a CD123-directed cytotoxin with human interleukin-3 (IL-3) fused to a diphtheria toxin, has been approved by the Food and Drug Administration (FDA) in treatment and remission induction therapy for adults with BPDCN. Tagraxofusp has produced promising overall response rates (90%) in patients with BPDCN. In patients with leukemia, circulating malignant cells may seed to the skin, particularly at sites of trauma as in our patient; our understanding of BPDCN's predilection for cutaneous tropism is poorly understood. In the setting of presentation of deep purple tumors, BPDCN should be considered a possibility CD123 staining is extremely helpful and can increase diagnostic certainty in those cases. It is essential to differentiate BPDCN from other mimics, including CD56+ AML, extranodal NK/T cell lymphoma, and CD8+ and $\gamma\delta$T-cell lymphomas.

References

Khan AM, Munir A, Raval M, Mehdi S. Blastic plasmacytoid dendritic cell neoplasm in the background of myeloproliferative disorder and chronic lymphocytic leukaemia. BMJ Case Rep. 2019;12(7).

Lee SE, Park HY, Kwon D, Jeon YK, Kim WY. Blastic plasmacytoid dendritic cell neoplasm with unusual extracutaneous manifestation: two case reports and literature review. Medicine (Baltimore). 2019;98(6):e14344.

Miedema J, Starr SR, Chan MP. Incidental diagnosis of blastic plasmacytoid dendritic cell neoplasm in skin excision for basal cell carcinoma. J Cutan Pathol. 2018;45(11):873–5.

Pemmaraju N, Lane AA, Sweet KL, Stein AS, Vasu S, Blum W, et al. Tagraxofusp in blastic plasmacytoid dendritic-cell neoplasm. N Engl J Med. 2019;380(17):1628–37.

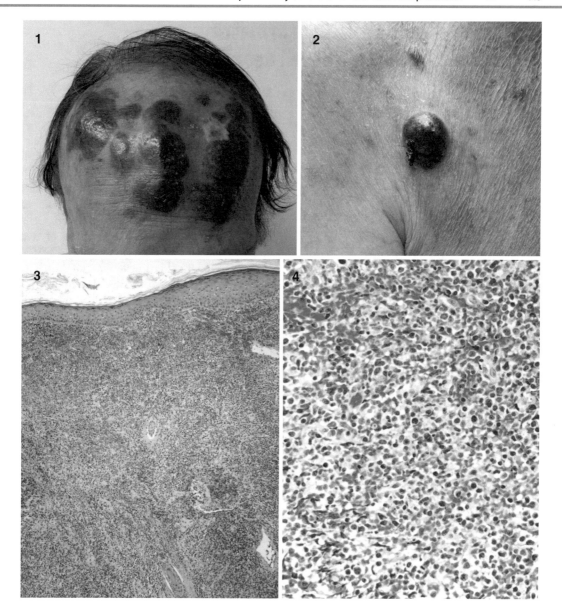

■ Fig. 1 Violaceous deep ulceration with punched out borders and surrounding deep purple edematous plaque on the frontal scalp. Published with kind permission of © Nicole LeBoeuf 2019. All Rights Reserved

■ Fig. 2 Deep purple plaque on the right upper anterior chest. Published with kind permission of © Nicole LeBoeuf 2019. All Rights Reserved

■ Figs. 3–4 Dense dermal infiltrate of intermediate sized mononuclear cells with irregular to folded nuclei, distinct to prominent nucleoli, and moderate amounts of eosinophilic cytoplasm, consistent with BPDCN. HE, ×10 (Fig. 3) and ×50 (Fig. 4). Published with kind permission of © Nicole LeBoeuf 2019. All Rights Reserved

Case 48. A solitary nodule of blastic plasmacytoid dendritic cell neoplasm in a young patient

J. A. Sanches and J. Cury-Martins

Age: 26   **Sex:** M

Clinical features: The patient presented with an asymptomatic dome-shaped, lobulated, erythematous tumor on the left superior back, with slow progressive growth for the last 6 months. No B symptoms, no evidence of clinical adenopathy, no comorbidities. Skin biopsy demonstrated a dense infiltrate of blastic cells through the entire dermis. Immunohistochemistry was negative for CD3, CD20, CD99, MPO, AE1-AE3, Melan-A, HMB-45, and desmin, with high KI67 and negative for TCR rearrangement (by PCR). Since no diagnosis was possible, the panel was extended with negative staining for CD2, CD7, CD8, TDT CD117, and EBV, and positive for CD4 and CD56. Flow cytometry of skin biopsy revealed cells positive for CD123/CD4/CD56/CD45, confirming the diagnosis. Laboratory tests revealed normal values of serum lactate dehydrogenase, b2-microglobulin, and blood count. Bone marrow biopsy and lumbar liquor puncture showed no involvement. PET-CT revealed the skin-only disease.

Diagnosis: Blastic plasmacytoid dendritic cell neoplasm (BPDCN) with skin-only, single lesion disease.

Follow-up: Patient was treated with six cycles of hyperCVAD with complete response, followed by allogenic hematopoietic stem cell transplantation (aHSCT), and is now on D+ 50 after HSCT, in complete remission.

Comment: BPDCN is a rare, aggressive hematopoietic neoplasm originating from plasmacytoid dendritic cell precursors, with overall survival of less than a year if left untreated. It has an incidence of 0.04/100,000 people and affects older males, with a 2–3.3:1 male to female ratio and a median age of 53–68. Cells should be positive for at least three of five markers: CD4, CD123, CD56, TCL1, CD303, and negative for other lineage markers such as CD3, CD20, CD34, MPO, EBV. The main sites of involvement are skin (60–100% of cases), bone marrow (60–90%), lymph nodes (40–50%), and CNS (30%). Many cases present with the skin-limited disease, but most of them will eventually develop disease progression with bone marrow infiltration. Regarding treatment, target therapies are being developed, with one anti-CD123 drug already approved by the FDA. When not available, more recent data support the use of an acute lymphoid leukemia-like regimen to prevent CNS spread, followed by allogeneic HSCT on selected cases.

References

Griffin GK, Togami K, Morgan EA, Lane AA. Developmental ontogeny of blastic plasmacytoid dendritic cell neoplasm (BPDCN) revealed by recurrent high burden clonal hematopoiesis, including in "skin-only" disease. Blood. 2018;132(Suppl. 1):2755.

Pileri A, Delfino C, Grandi V, et al. Blastic plasmacytoid dendritic cell neoplasm (BPDCN): the cutaneous sanctuary. G Ital Dermatol Venereol. 2012;147(6):603–8.

Sapienza MR, Pileri A, Derenzini E, et al. Blastic plasmacytoid dendritic cell neoplasm: state of the art and prospects. Cancers (Basel). 2019;11(5).

Venugopal S, Zhou S, El Jamal SM, Lane AA, Mascarenhas J. Blastic plasmacytoid dendritic cell neoplasm-current insights. Clin Lymphoma Myeloma Leuk. 2019;19(9):545–54.

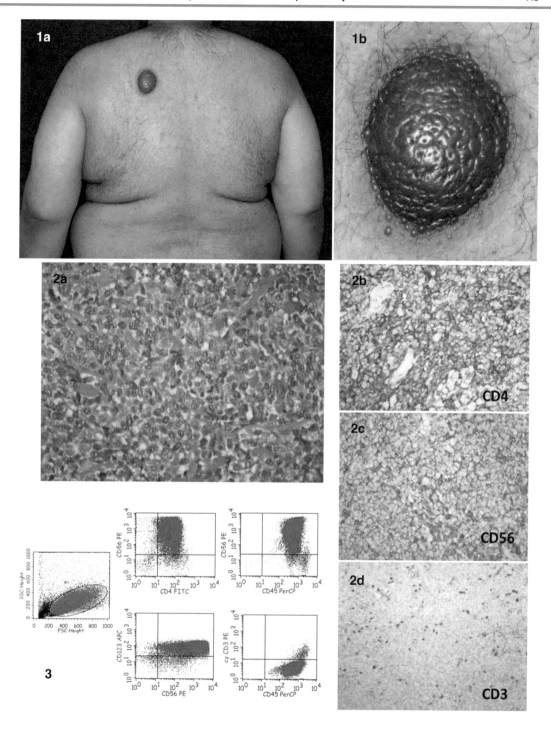

■ Fig. 1 (a) Dome-shaped, lobulated, erythematous tumor on the left superior back and (b) on a closer view

■ Fig. 2 Dense infiltrate of blastic cells through the entire dermis. (a) HE, ×40; (b) CD4, ×40; (c) CD56, ×40; (d) CD3, ×20

■ Fig. 3 Flow cytometry of skin biopsy revealing CD123+/CD4+/CD56+/CD3-cells

VI

Leukemias with the Secondary Skin

Case 49. Adult T-cell leukemia/lymphoma

K. D. Quint, R. Willemze, and M. H. Vermeer

Age: 68   Sex: M

Clinical features: A Moroccan descent with a week history of a progressive asymptomatic skin-colored infiltrated papules and nodules all over the body (with exception of the palms and soles). He had no other symptoms like fever, night sweats, or weight loss. Physical examination revealed enlarged inguinal, axillary and cervical lymph nodes. Laboratory investigations showed a mild leukocytosis (11.64×10^9/L; Ref 4.00–10.00), a hypercalcemia (4.58 mmol/L; Ref 2.15–2.55), and an elevated lactate dehydrogenase serum level (590 U/L; Ref < 248). A skin biopsy from the upper back revealed an atypical lymphoid dermal infiltrate consisting of pleiomorphic medium sized lymphocytes that showed epidermotropism with the formation of Pautrier microabscesses. Immunohistochemical staining showed a CD4+ T-cell with expression of pan T-cell markers CD3 and CD5, but complete loss of CD2 and CD7. Approximately 15–20% of the atypical cells expressed CD30. The proliferation index was high. Serological tests for HIV- and HTLV-antibodies revealed the presence of IgG antibodies suggestive for a HTLV-1 infection. External conformation with an immunoblot confirmed the HTLV-1 infection.

Diagnosis: Adult T-cell leukemia/lymphoma (ATLL), acute subtype.

Follow-up: PET-CT scan detected multiple enlarged and metabolically active lymph nodes in the inguinal, axillary and subcarinal area, but no bone marrow involvement. Treatment with combinations of vincristine, cyclophosphamide, doxorubicin, and prednisone (VCAP), doxorubicin, ranimustine, and prednisone (AMP), and vindesine, etoposide, carboplatin, and prednisone (VECP), demonstrated only minimal response. After three cycles complete chemoresistance occurred and three months later the patient died due to progressive disease.

Comment: ATLL is a rare T-cell malignancy caused by infection with the retrovirus human T-cell leukemia virus type 1 (HTLV-1). Infections with HTLV-1 are endemic in certain regions of Japan, South America, sub-Saharan Africa, the Caribbean region, Australia, and the Middle East. Approximately 2–5% of the infected individuals will develop an ATLL over time and can be classified in four subtypes, namely smoldering, chronic, lymphomatous, and acute subtype. HTLV-1 has a tropism for CD4+ cells, but can also infect CD8+ cells, B lymphocytes, monocytes, dendritic cells, and endothelial cells. While the smoldering and chronic ATLL subtype have a more indolent disease course, the lymphomatous and acute subtypes are known for their aggressive clinical behavior. Polychemotherapy or mogamulizumab (anti-CCR4) can be given as therapy, but the overall survival rate remains very poor. It was remarkable since Morocco was not an endemic area for HTLV-1.

References

Eusebio-Ponce E, Anguita E, Paulino-Ramirez R, Candel FJ. HTLV-1 infection: an emerging risk. Pathogenesis, epidemiology, diagnosis and associated diseases. Rev Esp Quimioter. 2019;32(6):485–96. Review.

Johnson W, Mishra A, Binder A, Gru A, Porcu P. Mogamulizumab versus investigator choice in relapsed/refractory adult T-cell leukemia/lymphoma: all four one or none for all? Haematologica. 2019;104(5):864–7.

Shimoyama M. Diagnostic criteria and classification of clinical subtypes of adult T-cell leukaemia-lymphoma. A report from the Lymphoma Study Group (1984–87). Br J Haematol. 1991;79:428–37.

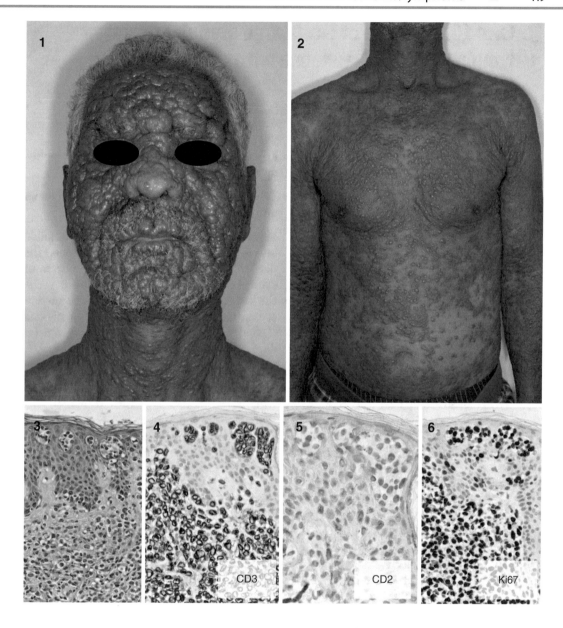

■ Fig. 1 Multiple red- to skin-colored non-ulcerating tumor on the face

■ Fig. 2 Symmetric monomorphic tumors on the trunk

■ Fig. 3 The atypical epidermotropic lymphocytic infiltrate with Pautrier microabscesses

■ Fig. 4 Positive CD3 expression on atypical cells

■ Fig. 5 Complete loss of CD2 on the atypical T-cell infiltrate

■ Fig. 6 The high expression of Ki-67 within the T-cell infiltrate

Case 50. A relapse of T-cell large granular lymphocytic (LGL) leukemia with chronic NK lymphocytosis in the skin

A. Bougrine, C. B. Hergott, O. K. Weinberg, D. C. Fisher, and C. Larocca

Age: 54   **Sex:** F

Clinical features: The patient with a history of T-cell large granular lymphocyte leukemia (LGL) and chronic NK lymphocytosis 9 years before the current presentation presented with multiple tender firm subcutaneous skin-colored to pink nodules on the lower legs in association with night sweats over a period of 2 months. Skin biopsy showed an atypical lymphohistiocytic infiltrate composed of small-intermediate-sized lymphocytes and infrequent large lymphoid cells in the dermis and subcutaneous tissue with extensive necrosis and angiodestruction. The lymphoid infiltrate was positive for CD3 and CD56. Two distinct populations of CD56+ and CD8+ T cells were abundant and collectively expressed TIA1, granzyme B, and perforin. EBV was negative by EBER staining. Laboratory investigations revealed an increased white blood cell count (8950 cell/mm³). Flow cytometry showed atypical T-cell large granular lymphocytes (CD2, CD3, CD5dim, CD7, CD8, CD57 positive) and reactive NK cells (CD2, CD7, CD8dim, CD16, CD56, CD57 positive), representing 10% and 41% of lymphocytes respectively. T-cell receptor (TCR) rearrangement showed an indeterminate peak with the Vγ9 primers (212 bp) in the skin and blood. PET-CT revealed FDG-avid foci in the skin, subcutaneous tissue, and intramuscular compartment of the lower extremities. Bone marrow biopsy showed an expanded NK population (17% of lymphocytes) and no T-cell clone.

Diagnosis: Recurrent indolent T-LGL leukemia and chronic NK-cell lymphocytosis.

Follow-up: At initial diagnosis the patient failed low dose methotrexate with prednisone. The disease was controlled with three courses of cyclophosphamide over the ensuing 8 years; the last dose was 5 months prior to the current presentation. At the present time, the patient is treated with pralatrexate 15 mg/m² given on days 1, 8, and 15.

Comment: LGL leukemias are rare lymphoproliferative disorders of mature T or NK cells with indolent and aggressive forms. STAT3 mutations are common in LGL leukemias, and STAT5B mutations are associated with aggressive disease. Autoimmune conditions and cytopenias are often observed. T/NK-LGL rarely involves the skin and may present with papules, nodules, ulcers, or telangiectatic lesions.

References

Duarte AF, Nogueira A, Mota A, Baudrier T, Canelhas A, Cancela J, et al. Leg ulcer and thigh telangiectasia associated with natural killer cell CD56(−) large granular lymphocyte leukemia in a patient with pseudo-Felty syndrome. J Am Acad Dermatol. 2010;62(3):496–501.

Lamy T, Moignet A, Loughran TP Jr. LGL leukemia: from pathogenesis to treatment. Blood. 2017;129(9):1082–94.

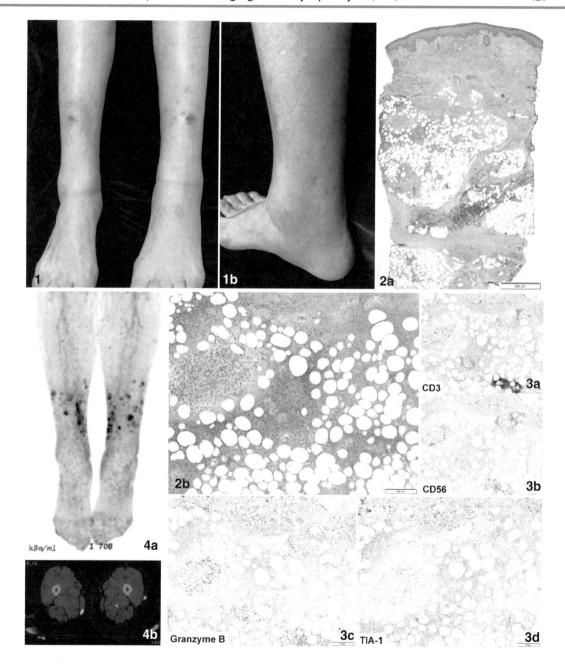

■ Fig. 1 Subcutaneous indurated erythematous nodules on the legs (**a**) and secondary scars (**b**)

■ Fig. 2 Dermal and subcutaneous involvement by a perivascular and interstitial lymphohistiocytic infiltrate with angioinvasion, angiodestruction, hemorrhage, and extensive necrosis. H&E, microscopic magnification 2× (**a**) and 10× (**b**)

■ Fig. 3 CD3 (**a**), CD56 (**b**), Granzyme B (**c**), and TIA-1 (**d**) expression on cytotoxic lymphocytes encircling vessels and infiltrating the dermis and subcutaneous fat. Immunohistochemical staining, original microscopic magnification 10×

■ Fig. 4 Multiple FDG-avid foci of malignancy in the soft tissue (**a**) and muscle (**b**) of the lower extremities

VII Other Lympho-

Case 51. Indeterminate dendritic cell histiocytosis

E. Akufo-Tetteh, B. Vydianath, and J. Scarisbrick

Age: 87 **Sex:** M

Clinical features: The patient with myelodysplastic syndrome with refractory cytopenia and multilineage dysplasia presented with a 1-year history of pruritic, tender, tumid erythematous papules, nodules, and plaques affecting the head, neck, arms, and upper torso. Secondary excoriations were noted along with low-grade lymphadenopathy along the cervical chain and a borderline enlarged spleen (13.5 cm). The laboratory tests were significant for elevated serum lactate dehydrogenase 297 IU/l (normal 135–225 IU/l), low platelet count of 51,000 cells/mm³ (normal 150,000–450,000 cells/mm³). HIV and HTLV 1 and 2 were negative. The skin biopsy showed heavy mild-to-moderate pleomorphic T-lymphocytic infiltrate with focal folliculotropism admixed with dense infiltrate of CD1a + Langerin- and S100-indeterminate cells with grooved nuclei. No large cell transformation, epidermotropism, syringotropism, or granulomas were identified on biopsy. Immunohistochemistry showed a CD4:CD8 ratio of 100:1 and small numbers of B cells. TCR gene rearrangement showed no distinct clone. The bone marrow showed reactive changes. PET/CT demonstrated diffusely scattered nodes in the neck, axillae, and mediastinum not exceeding 1 cm in diameter.

Diagnosis: Indeterminate dendritic cell histiocytosis.

Follow-up: Topical treatments were not effective. Localized electron beam therapy was not successful in controlling skin nodules. For that reason, TBSE was not pursued. Chemotherapy felt to be too risky because of underlying myelodysplastic syndrome. Currently, the patient is being treated with PUVA.

Comment: Indeterminate dendritic cell histiocytosis is a rare disease described in less than 50 cases thought to be caused by tissue-resident dendritic cells, which are en route from the skin to the lymph nodes. It presents mostly as skin lesions in adults and is often found in the presence of hematological malignancies. Diagnosis is based on the expression of both Langerhans cell markers (S100+ CD1a+) and non-Langerhans cells (CD68+), but not langerin (CD207). Treatment options are not standardized due to the rarity of this disease, but treatments such as surgical excision, radiotherapy, phototherapy, and methotrexate have been described. Chemotherapy and TSEB in more aggressive cases have been reported with some success, but reserved for cases involving more 50% of body surface areas.

References

Caputo R, Marzano AV, Passoni E, et al. Chemotherapeutic experience in indeterminate cell histiocytosis. Br J Dermatol. 2005;153:206–7.

Facchetti F, Pileri SA, Lorenzi L, et al. Histiocytic and dendritic cell neoplasms: what have we learnt by studying 67 cases. Virchows Arch. 2017;471:467.

Fournier J, Ingraffea A, Pedvis-Leftick A. Successful treatment of indeterminate cell histiocytosis with low-dose methotrexate. J Dermatol. 2011;38:937–9.

Horna P, Shao H, Idrees A. et el. Indeterminate dendritic cell neoplasm of the skin: A 2-case report and review of the literature. J Cutan Pathol. 2007;44(11):958–63.

Ishibashi M, Ouchi T, Tanikawa A, et al. Indeterminate cell histiocytosis successfully treated with ultraviolet B phototherapy. Clin Exp Dermatol. 2008;33:301–4.

Malhomme de la Roche H, Lai-Cheong JE, Calonje E, et al. Indeterminate cell histiocytosis responding to total skin electron beam therapy. Br J Dermatol. 2008;158:838–9.

Rezk SA, Spagnolo DV, Brynes RK, et al. Indeterminate cell tumor: a rare dendritic neoplasm. Am J Surg Pathol. 2008;32(12):1868–76.

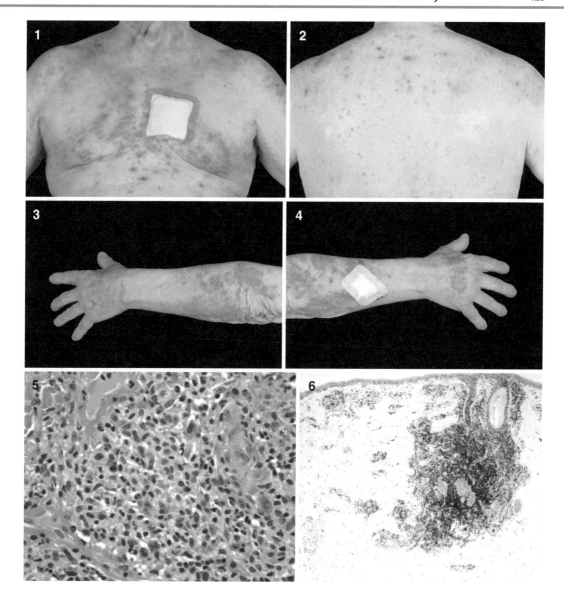

■ Figs. 1–2 Pruritic, tender, tumid erythematous papules, nodules, and plaques on the upper torso. Published with kind permission of © Julia Scarisbrick 2019. All Rights Reserved

■ Figs. 3–4 Coalescent erythematous papulonodules on the both forearms. Published with kind permission of © Julia Scarisbrick 2019. All Rights Reserved

■ Fig. 5 High power H and E showing neoplastic cells with bean shaped nuclei admixed with lymphocytes and eosinophils. Published with kind permission of © Julia Scarisbrick 2019. All Rights Reserved

■ Fig. 6 CD1 positive folliculotropic cells. Published with kind permission of © Julia Scarisbrick 2019. All Rights Reserved

Case 52. A unique presentation of hemophagocytic lymphohistiocytosis with ulcerating papulonodules

M. K. Collins, J. Ho, and O. E. Akilov

Age: 31   **Sex:** F

Clinical features: The patient with a history of benign seizures since childhood and asthma was hospitalized with fevers, abdominal pain, transaminitis, and leukopenia.

On a physical examination, there were ill-defined erythematous and violaceous dermal nodules, some with a collarette of scale scattered mostly on the lower legs, but also on the thighs, abdomen, and arms. Some nodules were ulcerated. Skin biopsy revealed a mild but diffuse dermal infiltrate of histiocytes with scattered intracytoplasmic erythrocytes. PAS, GMS, and Gram stains were negative for microorganisms. Infectious workup was negative for Hepatitis A, B, C, HIV, Rocky Mountain Spotted Fever, and Typhus. EBV and CMV IgMs were not elevated. An extensive rheumatologic workup showed mildly diminished C3, but normal C4. The initial bone marrow biopsy was unremarkable. Labs were significant for an elevated ferritin (>18,000 ng/mL), elevated triglycerides (>2000 mg/dL), low fibrinogen (78 mg/dL), and elevated soluble IL-2 receptor (>9000 U/mL). The patient continued to be febrile with transaminitis, which prompted a liver biopsy notable for erythrophagocytosis. Subsequent repeat bone marrow biopsy demonstrated hemophagocytic histiocytes.

Diagnosis: Hemophagocytic lymphohistiocytosis (HLH) with ulcerating papulonodules.

Follow-up: The patient was treated with systemic steroids and etoposide per the HLH-94 protocol (dexamethasone daily plus etoposide, cyclosporin, and intrathecal MTX in preparation for BMT). The patient developed pancytopenia, several bleeding episodes, and fungal pneumonia. Despite treatment with etoposide, the HLH progressed systemically, and she developed further ulcerations and erythematous nodules. After the continued progression of her disease, the patient decided to focus on comfort and died nine months after diagnosis.

Comment: HLH is a disorder in which overstimulation of the immune system causes organ damage due to the consumption of red blood cells, platelets, and other hematologic cells by macrophages. Two types of HLH have been described: primary HLH, which typically presents in children and is caused by genetic defects and secondary HLH, which may be triggered by infections (most commonly Epstein–Barr virus) or related to rheumatologic disease or malignancies (commonly lymphoid). Diagnostic criteria include either a molecular diagnosis consistent with HLH or five of eight of the following: fever, splenomegaly, cytopenias, hypertriglyceridemia/hypofibrinogenemia, hemophagocytosis in bone marrow, spleen or lymph nodes, low or absent NK-cell activity, elevated ferritin or elevated soluble IL-2 receptor.

References

Henter JI, Horne A, Arico M, Egeler RM, Filipovich AH, Imashuku S, Ladisch S, McClain K, Webb D, Winiarski J, Janka G. HLH-2004: diagnostic and therapeutic guidelines for hemophagocytic lymphohistiocytosis. Pediatr Blood Cancer. 2007;48(2):124–31.

Jun HJ, Kim HO, Lee JY, Park YM. Preceding annular skin lesions in a patient with hemophagocytic lymphohistiocytosis. Ann Dermatol. 2015;27(5):608–11.

Zerah ML, DeWitt CA. Cutaneous findings in hemophagocytic lymphohistiocytosis. Dermatology. 2015;230(3):234–43.

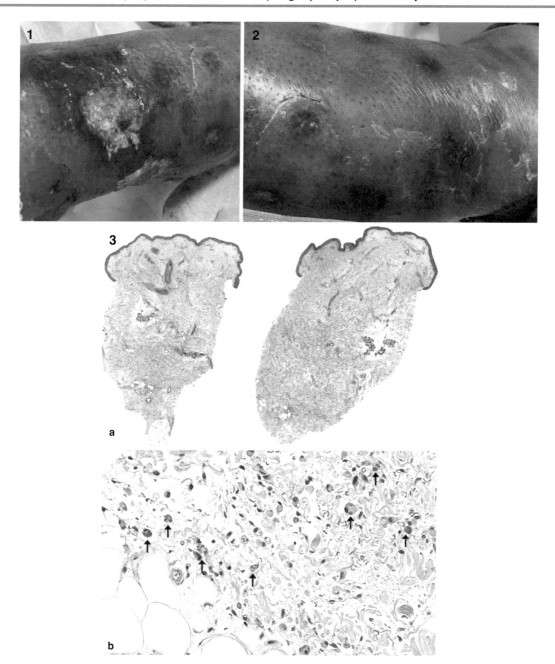

◼ Figs. 1–2 Erythematous and hyperpigmented papulonodules on the thigh and forearm

◼ Fig. 3 (a) Subtle predominantly histiocytic infiltrate in the deep dermis. HE, ×40. (b) Scattered hemophagocytic histiocytes (arrows), HE, ×40.

Printed in the United States
by Baker & Taylor Publisher Services